Every educator should have a copy of this book. [Ms. Tanner's] straightforward and sympathetic approach to finding a way out of a drug- and alcohol-induced nightmare gives me hope that meaningful lives for these young women can be rebuilt.

> —Donald S. Miller, M.A. Vice Chairperson; Communications Committee; California Teachers Association State Council

This is a very informative book that tells it like it is. I wish the mothers of the infants suffering from withdrawal on my unit could have had the chance to read it. This book could make a difference.

> —Jill A. Kamman, R.N. Neonatal Intensive Care and Pediatric Intensive Care Nurse

This book improved my awareness and compassion toward chemically dependent pregnant and parenting women. Fast reading, offers useful information, and hits the target!

> —Laurie James, author of *Outrageous Questions* and *Men, Women and Margaret Fuller*

# THE
# MOTHER'S SURVIVAL GUIDE TO RECOVERY
## All About Alcohol, Drugs & Babies

## Laurie L. Tanner

**NEW HARBINGER PUBLICATIONS, INC.**

Copyright © 1996 Laurie Tanner
          New Harbinger Publications, Inc.
          5674 Shattuck Avenue
          Oakland, CA 94609

Cover design by Laurie L. Tanner and Digital Graphics.
Text design by Tracy Marie Powell.

Distributed in U.S.A. primarily by Publishers Group West; in Canada by Raincoast Books; in Great Britain by Airlift Book Company, Ltd.; in South Africa by Real Books, Ltd.; in Australia by Boobook; in New Zealand by Tandem Press.

Library of Congress Catalog Card Number: 96-67937

ISBN 1-57224-049-0

First printing 1996, 5,000 copies

Dedicated to Sigrid, Jean, and Beth; for our Angel and Autumn; C, T.L., Kathleen, and Susan O.; and especially to the thousands of women and children who have touched me with their pain and their promise.

# Contents

# Foreword

*The Mother's Survival Guide to Recovery* is a book long waiting to be written. From urban disaster areas where cheap alcohol is consumed like soda pop and crack cocaine is king, to affluent neighborhoods where prescription drugs, high-grade cocaine, and vintage champagne are quaffed at elegant cocktail parties, pregnant women are becoming addicted and addicted women are becoming pregnant. Either way, the addicted mother's experience is too often an ordeal of shame and humiliation that frequently culminates in the birth of a baby bearing the dreaded stigma of its mother's disease.

"Get help, don't drink, and get on methadone if you're a heroin addict!" Good advice, but hard to follow if you happen to be pregnant, are in a psychological state that goes beyond despair, and have been rendered totally helpless by fear, shame, rage, and self-loathing. Ms. Tanner understands this paradox. She knows why addicts—in this case pregnant mothers—don't avail themselves of help even when they want it desperately. Through her clinical work with more than 2500 addicted mothers, she has come to know how it *feels* to be an addict. In solidarity with her clients she has permitted herself to experience the loneliness, desolation, and rejection of their lives. She has heard up close the anguished mantra of the addict/alcoholic: "I can't drink or drug, and I can't quit."

Despite some growing enlightenment in public attitudes towards addiction, a double standard still exists as far as women are concerned. Ms. Tanner tells us that "women live with society's disapproval [of their addiction] in a way that men rarely, if ever, experience." I think she is right. Addicted women tend to become objects of contempt in the eyes of most men and they are ostracized by other women. In the case of a pregnant addict, the double standard is tripled to include the fetus or the baby, and the mother's conduct is perceived as being tantamount to infanticide.

In recent years, negative attitudes like these have been amplified in society as a whole to form the basis of legislation which provides for punitive measures against addicted women during pregnancy or in the postpartum period. According to the American Society of Addiction Medicine's Public Policy Statement on Chemically Dependent Women and Pregnancy published in 1989 (see Appendix), "these measures have included the incarceration of pregnant women in jails to keep them abstinent, and the criminal prosecution of mothers for taking drugs while pregnant. . . ."

Although *The Mother's Survival Guide to Recovery* has been written primarily for addicted mothers, Ms. Tanner's insights and observations are also important for clinicians and therapists like myself who must struggle constantly with conflicted feelings evoked by the treatment process. In my own practice I have evaluated or treated about six pregnant addicts who were unable to stop drinking or using drugs despite adequate knowledge about the possible harm being done to their fetuses. Although I could empathize and feel compassion for the suffering of these women, I also felt contempt, disgust, and revulsion at their apparent lack of concern for human life. When feelings such as these arise in my relationships with patients, my training tells me to look elsewhere for their genesis. Even though I had not received any *formal* exposure to addictionology by the age of nine, I have a clear memory of feeling nauseous and frightened at the sight of my alcoholic and drug-addicted mother (whom I loved very much) slurring her speech and bumping into furniture during her pregnancy with my younger brother. Did she behave like this with me, I wondered? Eventually, my mother died from lung cancer brought on by a lifetime of alcoholic smoking, but her drinking disease lived on in me until I, unlike her, was blessed to find recovery. Once I realized that my impulse to reject these patients had been a manifestation of unresolved conflict between me and my mother about issues of *her* alcoholism during *my* pregnancy, my compassion returned, and I was once again able to adopt a fully caring stance in the treatment relationship.

The experience of contempt or similarly negative attitudes towards addicted persons signifies a failure to acknowledge the central truth of addiction: outside their awareness, addicts have *lost control* over their use of alcohol or other drugs and, as a result, will continue to drink or use compulsively despite adverse consequences to themselves or others *including* serious harm or even death for the fetus in the case of a pregnant addict. And they will hate themselves for doing it. Should we then collude with them by validating their self-hatred with punishment and contempt instead of acknowledging their suffering with treatment and compassion? Ms. Tanner repeatedly and brilliantly makes this cardinal point about loss of control in her book. Indeed, it is the single most important thing to remember when trying to understand the extent to which active addicts live with a sense of altered reality that is fundamentally different from what the rest of us experience in our daily lives.

*The Mother's Survival Guide to Recovery* carries a strong message of hope for addicted mothers who anticipate the arrival of their babies with foreboding and dread. Throughout her book, Ms. Tanner emphasizes the possibility of recovery and gently guides the reader towards the spiritual path whereby it may be achieved. She suggests practical ways for addicted mothers to overcome their natural resistance to recovery, and through words of encouragement at the end of each chapter always keeps them coming back to read the next one.

This book will expand our knowledge of pregnancy and addiction in a variety of important ways, and I believe it will save the lives of many who read it. While *The Mother's Survival Guide to Recovery* is not a medical or scientific book, its text rings with authenticity, and Ms. Tanner's careful research and consultation has avoided any serious errors. I hope it will be circulated widely as an invitation to recovery for addicted mothers everywhere, and as a must-read textbook for lawmakers, health professionals, clergy, and others who have the will and the spirit to work with this neglected population of suffering women and their innocent children.

All of us have had mothers of one sort or another, and many of us were given the chance to grow up with one. Ms. Tanner honors the obligation inherent in this sacred connection by refusing to abandon pregnant addicts as pariahs on the dungheap of conservative social reform. Instead, she gives them an unaccustomed pride of place as sick individuals with an incipient capacity for recovery, who therefore possess an ever-present potential to make a creative contribution to society—most notably the gift of a healthy child.

Garrett O'Connor, M.D.
Associate Clinical Professor of Psychiatry, UCLA
Past President of the California Society of Addiction Medicine

*Grateful acknowledgment to Dina Dire Brown and Lisa Rincon.*

# Introduction

## For You, Mom

I am so glad you are taking the time to learn about the problems faced when a pregnant or parenting woman is using drugs or drinking alcohol. You deserve to know the truth about what happens when alcohol and drugs are in your body, your baby's body, and in your life, family, and community.

I know, when you were a little girl, you did not dream of becoming addicted to substances that would hurt you and those you love, such as your children, family, and friends. I also know there is a reason each woman chooses to get high to handle the pain and confusion of her life.

This book was written to tell you the issues everyone will face when moms and children are impacted by alcohol and drug addiction. Mothers are the most important people in this deal. Why? Because pregnant women and mothers *can* change. Women can get help and support in order to become alcohol- and drug-free, to deliver healthy babies, and to be there to hold their children and care for them. When a mom drinks and drugs, certain consequences occur. As her life tumbles downward, the most important people in life, her children, will follow her there. Where? To more pain, guilt, confusion, denial, shame, separation, abandonment, self-punishment, and self-destruction.

*Don't let this happen to you! You are worth saving!*

It doesn't matter if you are fourteen years old or forty-four. It doesn't matter if you left school in the ninth grade, or finished several years of college. Whether you are black, beige, or brown, you can heal from the despair that drives your drug and alcohol use. If you were molested, assaulted, or damaged in any way, there are people and places who can and will help you. If a child has been adopted, an addict or an alcoholic can change her life and find peace. If your children are in foster care or in the custody of your relatives, you can find the courage to work toward reunification. Even if children were born with severe problems, you can improve their future.

Women get well whether they live in the projects, or on Miami Beach. It doesn't matter if a woman's skid row is her bedroom with mink coats in the closet, or hand-me-down clothes on a cot in a shelter. Women and their children get better even if dad is in jail, or still using, boozing, and cruising. Kids get better if mom is there for them—clean and sober.

I have worked with women whose families have been destroyed by chemicals. Whether rich, poor, or middle-class, the disease of addiction hurt every member of their family. Their own mothers or fathers drank or used drugs, or "turned them on" to an addictive lifestyle, or turned them into incest survivors. Being raped, beaten-up, or arrested is a common occurrence while women are copping (obtaining) their drugs and alcohol. Broken jaws, imprisonment, or a broomstick in the vagina is how some women have been hurt by the men in their lives. Prostituting for money or for alcohol and drugs have kept women homeless and abused by their dates.

Babies have been left with strangers for days, or have inhaled second-hand drug smoke while forgotten in the bedroom of a dope house. Children have been left in the care of child molesters, or grandparents who were old and sick. Women have hurt themselves, picking their skin apart, pulling out their hair, or burning in tattoos because they couldn't stop while under the influence or they couldn't deal with remembering what they did at last night's party.

Please keep going. . . . Read and learn . . . then act. This book will support your efforts to get your life together, to get well. You will be told about current concerns and future problems. You will learn what alcohol and drugs do to you and to your children, and become informed on how to get the help you want. You will read about the best ways to help your children get through their struggle with the effects of addiction, so they can be free to become happy in a healthier family.

You deserve to be shown the solutions to the problems you face. You have already started your new life by picking up this survival guide. Can you hear the applause? I am clapping and cheering and praying for your recovery, and for the happiness that will come to your family if you take baby steps toward becoming the mom you want to be.

A big part of you wants to get well, to be happy, to have a nice house for your kids, to show them how to solve problems, to be in a relationship where you are loved, respected, and valued. This is your future . . . if you recover from your addictions.

# CHAPTER 1

# What Is Happening?

This survival guide was written for the more than five million American women for whom drinking alcohol and using drugs has become a way of life—a way to cope with the confusion, pain, and frustration in a woman's mind, heart, body, and spirit. Mind-altering chemicals become the bridge she travels on in order to meet the world head-on, as she tries to find her place, her comfort zone, her worth.

Along the road to becoming an addict or an alcoholic, or both, life happens. Sex is a part of life. The religion of a woman's family, the culture she grew up in, and the role models she learned from usually did not prepare her to take care of herself before, during, and after sex. Many women with substance abuse problems have suffered sexual assault from males who were in and around their families while they were young. If you've been molested, hang in there and take heart, because you are not alone. Recovering, clean and sober women have spoken about and healed from the sexual abuse they have endured. You are a courageous person, and hope is on the way. Just keep reading.

A young woman's education about sex and how to avoid pregnancy is often from friends on the street, rather than from a knowledgeable, caring nurse or teacher. Education was found to be a determining factor in whether a woman used methods to protect herself from sexually transmitted diseases and pregnancy. Without adequate education, preparation, or confidence in herself, the man of the moment, or her husband, shows his desire for her and they join sexually. Maybe he introduced her to alcohol and other drug use during their relationship or before having sex.

The lovers don't talk very much—no birth control, no condom, no real plans for the future, no intention for her to become pregnant. They are not thinking about fatherhood or motherhood, for themselves or for each other. "Failure to prepare is preparing for failure" and an unplanned pregnancy will result unless ways to prevent conception are well understood, available, and used in every sexual encounter.

As women become sexually active, decisions about responsible lovemaking are often left to their male partners, or to fate. Many women believe they should not interfere with God's will in the area of reproduction. Their sex partners believe they have less responsibility than women in the matter of preventing pregnancy. Furthermore, young men frequently think that if "their" woman becomes pregnant, it is a clear measure of their manhood. But responsible parenthood will separate the real men from the boys.

It's difficult to prevent pregnancy while using drugs and drinking alcohol. Sometimes it's hard to believe you will still be alive in the next few years, or it's easy to feel "it can't happen to me," so why use protection against pregnancy or HIV? Although sex and drugs contain momentary relief from feeling bad, substance abusers still seek and need acceptance, security, and love. If a woman is chemically dependent, her alcohol and drug use will gradually increase, as well as the probability that she will become pregnant.

Love and hope in her life, she feels, will be found in the birth of an infant, regardless of her lifestyle, active addictions, sexual partners, or family problems. Having a baby can mean "I am somebody," "my baby will always love me," "I did what you wanted," or at least it will bring about change.

Addicted women and men discover they cannot make the positive life changes they want. The twists, turns, and crashes in their lives are controlled by their alcohol and drug use, rather than deliberate decision-making and family planning. As time goes on, abusing chemicals becomes the direction and the purpose of a drinker's and a user's daily life. It has become an addiction, a chemical upon which survival depends—a chemical dependency.

Both addicted and non-addicted parents feel that new life, in the birth of a baby, can make wonderful changes for them. However, serious problems emerge when the dark forces of alcohol and drug addiction are present inside a family with growing children, full of light, love, and demands.

Men can become willing to enter chemical dependency treatment when they see they'll lose their job, or already have. The wake-up call for women to deal with their substance abuse often occurs during pregnancy or the loss of their children. Professionals in perinatal addiction call this "a window of opportunity" because chemical dependency counseling can be most successful at this time in a woman's life.

Here is a word you will be hearing often—*perinatal*. Perinatal refers to those periods in a woman's life, usually between the ages of fifteen and forty-four, in which she is pregnant or parenting children. People who work with substance-abusing moms are experienced in dealing with the way addiction affects mothers, babies, children, and families, and can be referred to as perinatal addiction specialists.

No woman *ever* intentionally wants to hurt her baby. Intuitively, women know that alcohol and drugs are harmful to developing babies and children. For a substance-abusing pregnant or parenting woman, these two facts create feelings of hopelessness and helplessness—an enormous emotional and psychic crisis.

To recover from this crisis, women need appropriate support and effective treatment to become alcohol-free, drug-free, and the kind of mother they want to be. Almost four million women are pregnant each year. This book can comfort, educate, and motivate the estimated twenty percent of pregnant women who abuse substances in the United States. In 1992, one in nine women in California tested positive for drugs, including alcohol, at the time their babies were born. Therefore, more than 69,000 newborns in California, and up to 740,000 infants nationwide, had been exposed to harmful substances during prenatal development that year. These children will need helpful intervention, and clean and sober mothers, to grow into healthy, loving, emotionally secure women and men. Keep reading, and be one of them!

# CHAPTER 2

## Am I Addicted?

How does a woman know if she has a problem with drugs and alcohol? There are many ways to tell if you are becoming addicted to chemicals or if you are already addicted. You can be addicted even if you use once a month, twice a week, everyday, or only on payday. It doesn't matter how much you drink or use, when you use, what kind of drug, or if it's beer or liquor. What matters is . . . what happens to you and to your life when you get high?

## ABCs of Addiction

Inside you, these substances cause changes in your body, in your brain, and in your behavior. Some addicts and alcoholics feel physical effects while just thinking about booze and drugs, in anticipation of the high, like stomach butterflies, diarrhea, a pounding heart, or lightheadedness. Your body starts to depend on drugs and alcohol. When you stop you feel empty or sick—sweaty, vomiting, diarrhea, irritability, pain in muscles and joints, or wanting more (craving). These are some withdrawal symptoms alcoholics and addicts feel when their body is used to getting a chemical. It's called physical dependence.

You depend on alcohol and drugs to change how you're feeling and what you're thinking. In a lousy mood, bored, nervous, or afraid? A drink or drug changes your emotional and mental state. Chemically dependent people rely on drugs and alcohol to make themselves feel better, to stop negative thoughts, or to quit thinking so much. They can mentally, rather than physically, crave a substance and use it compulsively (bingeing). This is psychological dependence.

Over time, a drinker and a user will not be able to stop when they want to or when they need to. They cannot control when, where, with whom, or how much they drink or use, even when their lives are falling apart.

This is addiction. You physically, emotionally, or mentally *depend* on chemicals to continue living your life. You find you no longer have choices regarding alcohol and drugs, because the only thing you're doing is continuing to put them into your body. You have lost the ability to control or stop your drug use and your drinking.

Have you heard people talk about alcoholism or drug addiction as a disease, like cancer? Medical and chemical dependency treatment people define it as a disease because:

- it causes death (fatal)

- using drugs and alcohol grows into using *more* drugs and alcohol (progressive)

- it becomes the primary direction of an addict's and an alcoholic's life (obsession)

- if people in your family were addicted, you have a greater chance of becoming an addict or alcoholic, or both (genetic predisposition)

- it distorts your thinking, like refusing to believe that drugs and alcohol are a problem in your life (denial).

The good news is finding out you have it and getting the right kind of help can save your life and other lives from the diseased effects of addiction. More good news: you can get well from drug and alcohol addiction without surgery, it doesn't have to cost anything, and after you recover from this disease you might even feel okay about it, or even happy you had it.

Still have questions? Good. For answers, there are do-it-your-self questionnaires you can get from places like Alcoholics Anonymous and The Women's Action Alliance. A caring nurse, doctor, or treatment counselor can give you an easy screening test to help you decide. Examples of some questions are:

- Are you often permissive with your children because you feel guilty about the way you behaved while drinking? (For Women Only)

- Do you ever feel bad about your drinking? MAST (Michigan Alcoholism Screening Test)

- Did you ever think your father was an alcoholic? CAST (Children of Alcoholics Screening Test)

- Do you take pills to combat loneliness? (Questions About Prescription Drug Use)

If you are not excited about answering a questionnaire or calling someone you know who had a problem and are drug- and alcohol-free now, or talking to a doctor, nurse, or someone you trust, keep reading! You're doing great, and learning a lot.

## Warning Signs

There are some bright red warning signs in a woman's life that say stop! And she still drinks alcohol and uses drugs. People are substance abusers when painful, rotten things happen to them and negative situations come down in their lives, but they don't stop putting alcohol and drugs into their bodies.

To see if you are an addict or an alcoholic, or both, here's the story:

You tell yourself you're not going to drink or use today and you do anyway. A lot of your time and energy is focused on getting and using drugs and alcohol or recovering from a binge. Do you know what a twenty-four-seven is? (Using twenty-four hours a day, seven days a week). Perhaps you do not remember what happened while you were drunk or high, or don't know where your underwear went (blackouts). All your friends either drink or drug as much as you do, or more. Money for rent and food, as well as most of your cash goes to the liquor store clerk or to your dealer.

You may have become a sex worker, trading sex for drugs or booze, or sex for money for your drugs (or his drugs). A woman has a problem if she uses alcohol and drugs to escape pain, loneliness, or relationship problems. If you get into trouble with one drug, you switch to another, or have an alcoholic drink. Have you ever been arrested for drunk driving, possession, or being under the influence of an illegal, controlled substance?

Drugs and alcohol mess up your body by causing you to lose weight, gain weight, develop abscesses, high blood pressure, and nervousness; they ruin your teeth, give you heart, liver, stomach and reproductive organ problems. Are you losing weight? Have you stopped having periods or do you bleed a lot? Drugs and alcohol keep you awake when you should be sleeping, or they make you sleep too much. Chemicals damage the cells in your brain and in your nervous system, which changes the way you think, move, and respond to the world around you.

Have you forgotten to pick up your kids from your family or from the babysitter? If your children are being taken care of by someone else, or you're involved with child protective services, your drug and alcohol use probably played a part in this. Are you pregnant now and still drinking or using? Have you been beaten up, raped, or had your purse or car stolen while you were loaded or trying to get loaded? Do you know you have a problem, but continue to get high and tell yourself you don't have a problem?

Looking at your life, what has happened in your past, and what you have done, is really hard because you feel bad about it— guilty, ashamed, afraid, angry, and confused. Take it easy. Feeling really sad, depressed, and lost is appropriate, natural, and real if you are a woman who is chemically dependent. You have good reason to feel bad . . . it's a sad situation. I know it's been hard for you.

## What's Denial?

If you don't feel bad about what's happened in your life because of drinking and using, and you think you've answered questions about your life truthfully, keep reading! Drug and alcohol addiction is a tricky business ... and you've been tricked. All addicts and alcoholics have been deceived when alcohol or a drug is in their brain and in their lives, because it scrambles their thinking.

"I'm not that bad." "I only drink because of my boyfriend." "I just use because I'm stressed." "I can stop when I want to; I just don't want to." Chemically dependent people who explain their drinking and using like this cannot see what has happened in their lives as a result of abusing substances. They are honestly (not on purpose) deceiving themselves. Addicts and alcoholics want to believe that something (like life) or someone other than themselves is causing them to drink and use. If substance abusers can blame their lover, parents, or stressful life events, they don't have to feel as bad about themselves, or think it's their fault. They are denying that *they* have a problem with drugs and alcohol.

Guess what? It's not their fault. Denial is a mental distortion or twisted thinking that occurs when men and women drink alcohol and use drugs. Drugs and alcohol change how people understand reality and handle the day-to-day problems in their lives. What is real becomes unreal, untrue, and less painful. Addicts and alcoholics quit dealing with the facts of their lives because they are painful, and nobody enjoys pain.

If an addict and an alcoholic can stay in the dark about what's going on, they can keep getting high or drunk, and remain in the dark. Yes, it's become a closed circle of habits, frequent activities in their lives fueled by fear, denial, and chemicals. One way to think about "hitting bottom" with an addiction in your life is by realizing that you're drinking and using to handle the problems that booze and drugs have caused! People caught in the cycle of addiction will continue to suffer, as will their children and families. They cannot be the people they truly want to be.

Chemically dependent people want to protect their using and drinking because it is a solution, a way to cope with their inner life and outer circumstances. Now the solution (drugs and alcohol) has become a big problem, and denial keeps substance abusers from seeing addiction as the murderer it is. It kills the life force in women, men, and children. But, somewhere, inside of every alcoholic and drug addict, is a little voice that says "I shouldn't be living this way." If you are pregnant or a mother already, this little voice is turning into a scream.

The best way to know if you are chemically dependent is feeling way, way down, deep inside of yourself, that you want your life to be different—that your life *should* be different. You can't stop using and drinking, and you know you can't keep going on the way you have been. It is hard to imagine dealing with life without getting high, and it's become impossible to manage your life while drinking alcohol and using drugs. When you want to stop, and you can't, your life is really a living hell. If you are a mother or a mother-to-be, I know you would have quit using drugs and drinking alcohol before now, if you could have.

Not many people can quit using, boozing, and cruising on their own. Most men and women can and do stop being addicted, feeling addicted, and living addicted. How? When people get help and support, understanding and education, and the absolute truth about the disease of addiction they begin to change. Keep reading! It's a good thing!

# CHAPTER 3

# Using, Drinking, and Pregnancy

Women have fallen into abusing substances in an effort to make it through the pitfalls and challenges of their lives. Then a miraculous thing happens—they become pregnant. But now the miracle of having a baby turns into a nightmare if you are using drugs and drinking alcohol. Many substance-abusing women do not have a stable home of their own, family support, a place to go for medical care, transportation, or money. Even if a chemically dependent woman has money and other resources, she finds that her addictions keep her alone and isolated, unable to use the gifts she has to help herself or her baby. This chapter will show you how to find your way through the anguish of being chemically dependent and pregnant, toward a happy, healthy birth experience for both you and your baby.

## Letting the Secret Out

While working with more than 2500 pregnant and parenting substance abusers, not one woman told me she started using or drinking while she was pregnant. Drugs and alcohol were already in her life, and had been in her body before she was faced with a baby growing inside of her. So, first in her life were the chemicals, and second, the reality that she had conceived a child. It was too difficult, or perhaps unimportant, for a chemically dependent woman to stop drinking alcohol and using drugs before becoming pregnant. A perfect time to quit running and begin questioning your use of substances is now, instead of letting them run you! Pregnancy, while growing a new life inside of you, can be the beginning of a new way of living for you, too.

For a pregnant substance-abusing woman to start getting well, two conditions in her life must be brought out into the open: addiction and pregnancy. This is not an easy thing to do. She has tried to hide her addiction, and keep what has happened to her life as the result of using drugs and drinking alcohol a secret. Her secret is actually a huge, tremendously painful problem that has a lot of power. She lives with society's disapproval in a way that men will rarely, if ever, experience. In our society, it is less acceptable for a woman to drink booze or use drugs, even though women tend to use more socially acceptable substances and have less criminal involvement than men. Drunkenness and drug use is more permissible for men, tolerated by the community as manly, even necessary, conduct. Our culture is not as surprised when a male becomes alcoholic and drug addicted, and people seem less outraged when learning the effects that his addiction has upon his family.

Whether these beliefs are about sexual behavior or drug and alcohol use, we can understand how society's double standards for men and women *doubles* feelings of worthlessness, shame, and depression in a substance-abusing woman. If an addicted woman is pregnant, she will become even more isolated from her true self, her family, and her community as she suffers and crumbles under the judgment of this terrible social stigma.

A chemically dependent pregnant woman's secret has the power to destroy; but in the telling of the secret, healing will have already begun. Relief from living addicted can be just around the corner or on the next page. The truth will set you free and can give you the power to get help and support for your recovery from substance abuse.

# Accepting Pregnancy

By now, you have read some hard facts about drugs, alcohol, life, and society. Most women recognize that they have a problem with drugs and alcohol. Now let's go all the way. A substance-abusing woman needs to accept that she is pregnant in order to do good things for herself and her baby.

Nature has a sense of humor, but it's no laughing matter. During the first three or four months of a baby's development, a woman can be pregnant and not know it. When using drugs and drinking alcohol, it is hard to know if your stomach pain or vomiting is from morning sickness, a hangover, or chemical withdrawal. Feeling extremely tired is a daily problem, especially when coming down from a drug or a drink, and the possibility that you are pregnant is far from your mind. Mood swings, like being happy then crying for no reason, feeling trapped, depressed, and sad, are caused by changing hormones during pregnancy, as well as by booze and drugs.

Drugs and alcohol mess up your diet. Some addicts and alcoholics forget to eat, or feed themselves only once a day or once every few days. What, when, and how much they eat often occurs in the same way they binge on alcohol and drugs. The food they eat is usually not part of a balanced meal. Often it's fast food or whatever they can find in the kitchen or on the streets. It's hard for a female addict and alcoholic to know that her hunger sickness (not feeling hungry, wanting food all the time, knowing that she must eat right this second, cravings for certain foods) is due to being pregnant, rather than just another day of drinking alcohol, using chemicals, and eating on the run.

Some chemically dependent women have been hurting for so long in their emotional, mental, and physical lives that admitting they're pregnant is too much for them to comprehend. Like the denial that sets in when someone has a drug and alcohol problem, some women have been successful in refusing to believe that they are pregnant, especially if it's their first baby. They didn't choose to become pregnant at this time, their relationship is a mess, their families are far away or also have serious problems. All their energy goes into surviving the next twenty-four hours. Thinking of a newborn, or of becoming a mother, is just too overwhelming. With the help of drugs and alcohol, some substance-abusing women hope to change the reality of pregnancy by denying that it is real.

*Don't let this happen to you! You and your baby are worth saving.*

# If Your Partner Is Addicted

Whether you became pregnant on purpose or by accident, as a substance-abusing woman you will experience some strong feelings that can get in the way of your healthy recovery if you are not prepared for them. Understanding these emotions will help you make it through this tough time in your life. Most women must go through periods of grief, shame, and loss, which are especially hard if you are single. Or, perhaps you feel alone, because your husband, partner, or family member is speeding down the same road of addiction in his or her life, and cannot be there for you or help you in any positive way. If this person, whom you care for and who cares for you, is actively using drugs and drinking alcohol, his or her influence on you will not be a good one.

Many women have found out the hardest way imaginable just how damaging their relationship with a chemically dependent partner can be, especially if he is an intravenous drug user or participates in other risky activities. It's possible thousands of women don't know their man's drug history or perhaps they have ignored it. Maybe they don't even use drugs or alcohol themselves. But, without protection, they became HIV-positive. Women having the HIV/AIDS virus from sexual relations are the second largest female group to become infected, and their lives have been changed forever. *Believe* that you and your baby are entitled to protection.

If your life includes an addicted boyfriend, partner, or family member both of you have choices to make. Each person who is chemically dependent has to make the decision to change and take action to recover. All individuals must do it themselves. No one can do it for you, no one can do it for your loved one; but you're the only person who can do it for the baby inside you. Continuing to hang out with your drug-using and alcohol-drinking partners, even if it's your husband or loved one, will surely keep you sick and make your baby sicker.

Your partner has to handle his or her own addictive behaviors. As a pregnant alcoholic and addict, your responsibility is twice as serious and three times as hard. You have to carry both you and your baby toward recovery. Your job is tough enough and you'll need all your energy to get well. Sometimes it comes down to a heartbreaking choice—your baby or your addicted partner.

Allow your loved ones to do what they have to do: keep getting high or get the help to change. It's their choice. The death grip that alcohol and drugs can have on someone's life cannot be loosened by anyone but themselves. Taking care of yourself by removing yourself from dangerous using and drinking situations gives other addicted people the space they need to make a decision toward light or addictive darkness. This is a very loving thing to do for your chemically dependent partner. Find the courage and the strength inside of yourself to let go of people who cannot support you and your baby's welfare. I know these are not easy choices for you or for your partner. Your decision does not have to be forever; just do it for yourself and for your baby, right now. And wait and see. Life is always changing, and your relationship with significant others can change, hopefully for the better. Be patient, and do what you know is right. Let 'em go—to keep your baby healthy and yourself drug- and alcohol-free.

## You Are Number One

You have needs now, and you are entitled to have these needs met, and it does not depend on you being a perfect person. Women will usually blame themselves not only for their own problems, but for other people's problems, too. We feel we are the source of most of the difficulties that surround us, even those over which we have little control. If a substance-abusing woman feels good or tries hard and succeeds, she will often think it was due to luck or she has escaped being found out. If she experiences failure, she can feel overly responsible, entirely guilty, and defective. We tend to think problems in life are due to something inside of ourselves that is broken, or something that we are missing. Chemically dependent women believe "I don't do enough, I don't have enough, I am not enough." This leads women to feel shameful, and believe they are helpless and powerless to change their lives, because it feels hopeless to try to change ourselves. You are more than the bad things you feel you are; you are more than shame. You are human, and you will change as life goes on. Let's make sure those changes are good ones, full of hope instead of shame, as your baby is growing inside of you.

Losing something or someone precious to you causes grief and mourning. Everybody has lost something, so everyone has experienced grieving; it is a natural, normal human reaction. There is shock, anger, denial, and incredible sadness in letting go or losing someone or something you loved and needed, or thought you needed.

It's a sad realization that drug and alcohol dependency can get in the way of anyone's parenting. Substance-abusing women want to protect feelings of being good moms because this is so important for most women's self-image and emotional survival. But every mom has doubts about how she treats her child. It's hard to see that we don't always act like the mother we think we are, and harder to admit that we need some help. Becoming the best parent you can starts with an ache. A grieving process usually occurs when people accept that they are addicted, and realize that they have lost feelings of self-worth and self-respect, as well as the love of their families, because of drugs and alcohol. But, *losing something or someone does not mean you are a loser!*

Having to rely on substances to make it through life can produce feelings of hopelessness, failure, even a desire to die. Living your life drugging and drinking can make death seem like a solution, but it's just another trick. Addicted people want relief. I spell relief: r e c o v e r y.

By getting chemical dependency treatment and support, you can get through feelings of grief, loss, depression, and hopelessness. It will become safe to be who you are, and it'll be okay to feel good and bad feelings. Expressing how and why you hurt is part of the getting-well process. If you begin your recovery, you will survive the painful emotions of accepting that you are a person with an addiction problem and you will end up feeling good about yourself.

There is a very special kind of grief, a horrible fear of loss, that substance-abusing pregnant women carry inside their hearts.

This is the heavy terror that your baby will be taken away from you because of your drug and alcohol addictions. Just like a lioness, a human mother will fight to keep her infant close to her at almost any cost. But lions do not drink alcohol or use drugs. Since we are human beings, we need to walk through the jungle of fear and not let its terror keep us frozen in the dark and powerless, especially if someone has already lost a baby through losing custody or through death. The time to start fighting for your future, and your baby's future, is while you are pregnant. If you want to win this battle and not lose the baby who is in your heart and in your body, you need to know who or what the *real* enemy is.

## Unmasking the Real Enemy

Other people are not the enemy if you are pregnant and need to get clean and sober. Sometimes a woman's drinking and drugging makes her believe that clinic, hospital, or doctor's office personnel are the enemy. Perhaps she has talked to a healthcare person about her substance abuse, and they were not kind, supportive, or knowledgeable about chemical dependency. Many substance-abusing women want to think it is their partner's fault that they cannot stop using or drinking. If child protective services are in your life, it is easy to believe that your case worker, dependency court judge, or investigator are enemies working against you, particularly if you have had painful, punishing experiences with them in the past, or have heard terrible stories from other women.

Maybe your relatives or neighbors, who can't mind their own business, become your enemies when they talk to you about your alcohol- and drug-using lifestyle. If you have been in treatment for your drug addiction and alcoholism before, maybe the treatment counselor's office or the recovery home feels like enemy territory. If you have warrants or probation violations, police officers and other criminal justice people can seem very threatening to you, with good reason. However, if you have court dates pending, don't let your legal situation stop you from getting the help you need and want. A pregnant woman is recognized as a responsible person if she is receiving prenatal care and substance abuse treatment.

Drugs and alcohol are the true enemies of healthy moms, babies, and children. If alcohol and drugs are in your body, that is where the problem is. Getting drugs and alcohol out of you is simple, but not easy. First you have to stop using and drinking.

Some women need a lot of help to stop. Often they must detox so that withdrawing from chemicals won't hurt them or their babies, especially if they are addicted to alcohol or narcotics (heroin, codeine, prescription drugs). Chapter 8 will explain how to get help for detoxification and other forms of treatment. But the solution is still the same—get help to stop exposing your baby to chemicals. *You can do this.* I know you can because I believe in you. I believe in your goodness that drugs and alcohol tried to snuff out. It's there inside of you, right now. Tap into it.

Here is the honest truth, and you can make it your own. The most important, caring thing you could wish for is that your baby has a good brain and a healthy body with which to begin life. This fact, to me, is more important than what could happen after the baby is born. Pregnant addicted women have pressure, a timetable that can feel like a time bomb. There are less than nine months for an infant's organs and nervous system to fully develop. This means getting treatment for you and your baby is urgent, and cannot wait for anything or anyone. Once the baby is delivered, we cannot go back in time or put the baby back inside of you to change or improve oit's development. Nothing can replace a healthy womb for a baby's growing stages of mind and body.

Many alcoholic and drug-using women have experienced problems in the way their body handled pregnancy. The main life support system for a baby is mom's placenta and umbilical cord. Chemicals, especially cocaine and methamphetamine, have been found to cause the placenta to separate (abruption of the placenta) or plant itself too low in the uterus (placenta previa). If you are chemically dependent, you are at risk for ruptured membranes, hemorrhaging (bleeding), and contractions which can cause pre-term labor and a premature delivery.

If a baby is born with severe problems, your hope of a happy life with your baby will quickly fade. Life with a sick baby focuses on the infant's struggle for survival, and is not the gentle, loving bonding time you expect to have with a new baby. Other difficulties can arise even if newborns show little or no signs of withdrawal or other problems, but their mothers used drugs or drank alcohol during pregnancy. A second painful reality is that difficulties can become evident when children are a year old, or two or three, or ten years old. No mother wants her child to start kindergarten and not be able to sit still, listen well, or get along with the other kids. And if the mother still drinks alcohol and uses drugs, each child's problems will continue and multiply. An unhappy, stressed-out child cannot do a good job at school or at home.

Your fear that other people, especially authorities like a doctor, family member, case worker, or probation officer, will find out that you are pregnant and abusing substances, can keep you from saving your baby's life. Please, don't let your fear of discovery stop you from giving your baby what he or she needs most—a good brain and a healthy body. Let's make sure you and your baby are healthy before, during, and after delivery.

Most women hope for a good life with a loving partner and beautiful, healthy, well-behaved children. When it looks like this dream isn't going to come true, it causes waves of confusion, pain, and grief. Your life hasn't turned out the way you wanted it to. Lost hopes and unfulfilled dreams of the perfect family can hurt women and mothers. Don't let grief eat away at you any longer. It's okay to let go of your idea of a perfect family and not let anything or anybody keep you from what you want now—a healthy baby in your arms, and to live a good life, without alcohol and drugs to tear it down. There is no greater victory or better job that you could be admired for than changing your life for the sake of your baby.

No matter how far along you are in your pregnancy, it is *never too late* for a woman with substance abuse problems to get help. You can do it. There are two actions you need to take that will help you and your unborn child: (1) get prenatal care and (2) get help and support to become clean and sober. You could do it now! Good work, mom, and keep reading.

# CHAPTER 4

# Prenatal Care:  Get It
# Because You Care

Let's spell out what every pregnant woman needs: prenatal care. Natal means birth. So prenatal care is medical attention that is needed from the time a woman conceives until the baby is born.

## Where To Find Prenatal Care

Women need prenatal care especially if they are drinking booze and using any drugs, even if those drugs have been prescribed by a doctor or have been given to you by a friend or relative. Go to a doctor, clinic, or hospital for prenatal care. There are some good, progressive hospitals and women's healthcare facilities that have special OB (obstetric) clinics for substance-abusing women. These clinics can really be a lifesaver for you and for your baby. The doctors and nurses are experienced and usually very supportive when they work with chemically dependent pregnant women. Often, there are more female doctors and nurses who work in special OB prenatal care and women's specialty clinics. They try to make you feel more comfortable, especially if you've been hurt by incest or sexual abuse. Many private physicians and managed healthcare companies accept substance-abusing women, low income families, and Medi-Cal or Medicaid recipients. Just find someone you can be honest with, someone who will be honest and helpful to you, and somewhere that is close by so you can get to your appointments as often as necessary and on time.

Doctors and nurses who are experienced and specially trained to work with pregnant women who used or drank during pregnancy can do a better job for you and your baby. They know what to look for in pregnant moms and developing babies who have been exposed to drugs and alcohol. So if a problem arises, they will know what to do and they will do it sooner than a medical professional who is not specifically trained or experienced in perinatal addiction. And if a perinatal specialist doctor or nurse tells you they do not see any problems after your prenatal care checkup, you will feel better and have more peace of mind because they know what they are talking about.

Doctors, nurses, treatment counselors, case managers, and others are just like anybody else. If they did not have the specialized education, a clear understanding of addiction, or much experience in working with pregnant and parenting substance abusers, they would not be able to give you the most effective care. We have already read about how drug addiction and alcoholism is a tricky business for women. It's not easy for the professionals who want to help them either.

The best ways to get help are to: educate yourself, which you are already doing by reading this book, and find the courage to talk about your problems. Meet with medical and treatment professionals who know how to support you, and can give you and your baby the best they have to offer. After all, you are letting go of your secret and bringing good things into your life like prenatal care. This is something for you to feel good about, and something other people should support.

It is okay to ask a doctor, nurse, or counselor if they have worked with pregnant and parenting addicts and alcoholics before. It is really okay to ask if you can see a doctor or counselor who has had special training in perinatal addiction. It is also okay to ask for a female doctor or counselor if it would make your prenatal care and substance abuse treatment less stressful for you. Finally, it is more than okay to find the best people you can to help you win the battle of addiction and have a healthy newborn baby. You have every right to ask!

If you had a rotten experience when you tried to get prenatal care before or when searching for your place in a recovery program, does this mean you should forget about obtaining these services? No way. If you went somewhere for help, and you feel you were not respected or were mistreated, you must keep going. You must keep working to accomplish your goal—to get good prenatal care and help and support to be clean and sober. This help could be recovery in a treatment program and twelve-step meetings, moving out of your using environment, and talking to someone experienced in addiction about your feelings.

Addicts and alcoholics don't let anything or almost anyone get in their way when they need drugs and alcohol. This means chemically dependent people have a lot of willpower to get what they want and make things happen. Go after what you need and deserve—prenatal care and drug and alcohol treatment—the way you struggled to get high. It's okay to ask for what you want. You are different now by choosing to make positive changes in your life, and good things will happen for you.

Sometimes you just gotta hang in there, even if the healthcare clinic or the treatment program isn't exactly what you thought it would be. Just find the people and the places that give you what you need—effective treatment, for your health and for your addictions. You and your baby are absolutely worth it.

You can get well, and you don't even have to like it! Isn't that great? You do not have to be "Mary Sunshine" or feel good all the time or act "good" to get the help you want. You can get the support and treatment you need by showing up and being on time for medical appointments and treatment groups; by being cooperative, even if it's painful, like talking honestly about your life and addictions to a nurse or counselor; by following the directions that medical and treatment people ask you to follow, like taking medicine at the correct time or going to a recovery meeting in your neighborhood; and by taking the plunge—tell your story, let your problems out! You stood on a mountaintop in your life, your addictions pushed you off a cliff, and now you can fall into a prenatal care clinic and a drug and alcohol program instead of landing in the garbage dump. Now that's a good thing!

Many women feel suspicious or afraid when they visit a doctor's office, health clinic, or hospital for a checkup. Understanding what healthcare professionals need to do to give a thorough examination helps women feel less fearful and more in control about what is happening in their body and in their baby. Nobody likes putting their feet in the stirrups of the exam table or their arm on the chair support for blood work. If you are prepared for what will happen next, you will feel more confident when doctors, nurses, laboratory technicians, midwives, and others begin medical procedures.

Feel free to ask questions and be sure to listen for the answers. This is your party, your prenatal care experience. These procedures, some of which are listed below, are absolutely (no fooling) necessary to insure your baby's health and to follow his or her development.

## Prenatal Procedures

A nurse will probably talk with you to obtain your medical history. You will be asked if you or any of your relatives have had certain diseases, like German measles (rubella) or diabetes. Are you allergic to any medications? Explain any surgeries, the number of pregnancies, and what happened with these pregnancies. A lot of women have had children, miscarriages, therapeutic abortions, and other incidents that are important for the nurse to know about in order to get an idea of what your body has been through. It is very helpful for her to know any problems you've had with other pregnancies, and labor and delivery experiences.

You will be asked when your last period was. Try to be as exact as you can because the nurse and doctor will use this date at the beginning to judge how long your baby has been growing. Let the cat out of the bag regarding your drug and alcohol use during the past year. This information will tell a healthcare professional where and what to look for in terms of your health and the health of the baby.

If you change doctors or prenatal care clinics during your pregnancy, be sure to ask that your medical records be sent to where you are receiving prenatal care now. When you request your prenatal care records, the nurse or office person will ask you to sign a release of information. This gives your permission for the healthcare provider to send your confidential medical records where you want them—to the doctor or OB clinic that is currently taking care of you. Help the doctor, nurse, or midwife to better track your baby's growth and how your body is managing a developing baby. It is one of the responsible, loving things you can do when you are pregnant. Doing things like this, caring enough to request and sign a release so you can have good, continuous medical care, will help you feel better about yourself and your pregnancy.

Any woman who has used drugs or alcohol during pregnancy is considered to have a high risk pregnancy. This means there are special things that you, your doctor, and your nurse need to watch out for. Don't let this scare you. Any woman over thirty-five years old also has a high risk pregnancy simply because of her age. High risk pregnancies mean there is a greater likelihood that some problems could come up. By getting prenatal care, you are helping your pregnancy to be in a lower, high risk category. Keep reading, you're doing a good job! And if you are already getting consistent prenatal care, you're doing a great job.

How soon should a pregnant woman begin prenatal care? The best answer to this question is as soon as humanly possible. Remember that prenatal means the whole time before birth. Pregnancy is broken down into three stages of your baby's development. This stuff is really important to know because different structures in a baby, like the brain or the bones (skeletal system), develop at different times.

## The Three Stages of Pregnancy

The first trimester begins with the fertilized egg growing to three inches in fourteen weeks. Stomach, intestines, mouth, and the "food tube" (gastrointestinal tract) are the earliest organs to form. Then the brain, nerves, sex organs, kidneys, respiratory system, and heart develop and may begin to function. The heart beats, the brain and nerves are active, even some muscles contract in the baby's body. The fetus' face, eyes, bone mass (skeleton), arms, legs, teeth, fingernails, and toenails are also present.

A lot of body parts were created in a short time since the egg and sperm did their dance. Because so many important organs begin growing and expanding in the first three months, the fetus is very vulnerable to the effects of drugs and alcohol, and is therefore more easily harmed.

The second trimester is the middle stage of a child's development inside mom's uterus. Between fourteen and twenty-seven weeks the baby grows rapidly as the cells increase in number and get bigger to form tissue in the organs and the body. The sex organs can be identified, the liver begins working, and blood cells form inside the bones' marrow. The skin is completed, and its waxy covering for an easier delivery is there too.

Now the fetus is called a baby, who can kick, hear sounds, suck a thumb, and grow hair. The baby is now bigger than your foot! Organs, like the brain and intestines, are functioning better as the baby grows to twelve inches, and are less susceptible to problems than in the first trimester.

The third trimester, twenty-eight to forty weeks of growth, is the last three and one-half months of a baby's development. The baby is gaining weight and needs to add about three pounds in three months. This is another vulnerable time if mom is drinking or using. The baby begins to store iron, calcium, and other nutrients from mom's bloodstream in order to continue growing. The baby can move energetically or cry weakly, and gets thicker skin, becoming plump. Delicate, complex structures like the ears and nose finish developing.

If born prematurely, the baby hasn't gotten to fully develop where it was supposed to—inside mother's womb. A baby can survive if born early in the last trimester or maybe earlier, but would have to remain in the hospital to gain weight and receive treatment for any health complications.

Now you will know what trimester you are in when the healthcare person tells you how many weeks along you are in your pregnancy. And you'll know the bottom line about drug and alcohol use during pregnancy. You will know which areas in an infant's body could be most disturbed from drug and alcohol exposure at a given time. Medical specialists can tell us that most prenatally exposed children are not born outwardly deformed, but that they frequently have specific behavior problems and nervous system disorders as newborns and while growing up.

# Preparing for the Prenatal Exam

Some women tend to have higher blood pressure from the massive amount of hormones produced during pregnancy. The nurse or doctor will take your blood pressure at every visit, wrapping a cuff around your upper arm and reading the amount of pressure it takes for your heart to keep blood moving through the tubes, called blood vessels, to all parts of your body.

This is something to watch for because the blood vessels, which carry food calories to nourish your body, can become tight. The blood vessel tube is smaller, constricted. Therefore, less blood and less nourishment is getting to the areas that need it most for a baby to grow. Blood is life. It is desperately needed to build new tissue in the placenta, the uterus, and the baby. Drug and alcohol use increases blood pressure by tightening, constricting the vessel, which decreases the flow of blood. Some of the drugs that cause this are caffeine (coffee), amphetamine or methamphetamine, alcohol, and cocaine.

Low blood pressure can be temporary, like when a woman lies down and her uterus is putting pressure on several large blood vessels in her pelvic area. When she gets up, she might feel dizzy or her heart might pound. Her blood flow will quickly return to normal. Less often, it signals weak nerves or anemia.

You will be weighed at every prenatal care visit. Calories are turned into energy quicker and used up faster when you are pregnant, so you need more calories. This is why eating enough and eating the right food is so important. It is vital for your nurse and doctor to know how much weight you are gaining; that is, if you are underweight, or weigh too much, for that stage of pregnancy. If you need help to gain or lose weight, your doctor or clinic nurse should have a nutritionist talk with you to suggest the right foods for you to eat and discover the foods you like.

Special problems require creative solutions, so get the most useful information from every person you talk to. For example, some women's temporary homes do not have a refrigerator, so a nutritionist can tell you what foods would be nutritious yet would not need refrigeration. The nurse and doctor watch for extra water in your tissues, such as swollen ankles or hands.

The nursing professional will take your temperature orally (by mouth) at each visit. Fevers increase the rate at which your body uses up calories and will raise your blood pressure. Fevers can also signal if your body is fighting an infection which can harm the baby.

Most prenatal care practitioners will give you a TB skin test at your first visit to see if you have been exposed to a disease called tuberculosis. TB germs are sprayed through the air by people who have the disease in their lungs or throat, so it's easy to become exposed to it. The nurse uses a small needle to put a little liquid, called tuberculin, under the skin of your forearm. A health worker must look at the place on your arm in two to three days to see if you have had a reaction and have been exposed, or if you are clear. If you are positive for TB, you may need medication. Get the TB skin test to make sure you're okay.

Laboratory tests are really important. Urine and blood tests, especially at your first visit, tell the healthcare professional how your body is functioning. Blood tests are necessary to find out your blood type and check for toxemia (blood poisoning from bacteria), anemia (not enough red blood cells), and other diseases.

I know, I hate needles too. You can help yourself get through the tests that every pregnant woman needs to have. When the lab technician has to take your blood, close your eyes and use your imagination. Think of pleasant thoughts—a horse galloping across a field, a dolphin playing in the ocean's waves, or your favorite song from the radio.

Your blood will show if there are illnesses your doctor needs to treat. Testing for sexually transmitted diseases is very important, because thirteen million people catch at least one every year. Women can have a problem, like syphilis, chlamydia, or gonorrhea, and not know they've been infected unless their doctor tests them. Some diseases are easily treated with medication and some need lots of medical attention so you can be in the best possible health during your pregnancy. One thing is certain: if you do not get the medical care you need, these infections can injure your baby, causing birth defects, blindness, pneumonia, or inflamed brain tissues.

Almost all hospitals, OB clinics, and responsible doctors now test for the presence of drugs and alcohol in pregnant women. *Don't hit the panic button.* First, simply by reading this book you have started treatment by educating yourself about addiction and pregnancy. Second, nobody gets well if they have the disease of drug addiction and alcoholism and it remains a secret. Third, good prenatal care would not be good or beneficial if something harmful, like infections, alcohol, or drugs, are in your body, and the doctors and nurses did not do everything they could to help you. They would have neglected you and your baby's health and well-being.

Too many people have neglected you in too many ways. Now you can take better care of yourself and your baby. If you have a positive drug and alcohol test while pregnant, your healthcare providers will talk to you. They need to know if you are getting chemical dependency treatment, or are ready and willing to get it. They should give you drug and alcohol education literature, and point you in the right direction for whatever resources you need. These referrals can include quality treatment programs, childbirth and parenting classes, counseling, childcare, and social services (Aid to Families with Dependent Children; Women's, Infant's, and Children's Nutrition Program, housing advocates, and so on). Healthcare professionals should make sure that every pregnant and parenting substance abuser feels safe enough to get prenatal care and the referrals she needs to get well and help her family.

Pelvic, abdominal, and breast exams are usually done at the first prenatal care visit. Your medical examiner checks the size of the birth canal, the condition of the cervix, and looks for any out of the ordinary discharge. By giving you an abdominal checkup, the doctor or nurse learns the size of your uterus and the baby's position inside.

A breast exam is also important to make sure you have no lumps or nipple discharge, and to talk about the possibility of breast-feeding. Please consider breast-feeding if there is no medical reason why you shouldn't. Breast milk is recommended as the ideal food for infants. It provides great protection for your baby against illnesses, allergies, infections, and stomach and bowel problems. Infants will get the right amount of nutrition, at the correct temperature, available at a moment's notice, and prepared with love! Both moms and babies benefit from the close contact, and the price is right. Breast-feeding can be a sweet incentive to stay alcohol- and drug-free, and there are supportive health workers who can show you how.

Other tests are more exciting for a pregnant woman, such as an ultrasound sonogram. Sound waves from the technician's equipment are directed at the abdomen and echo back to form a visual picture of the baby's body and where the baby is precisely located inside the womb. Your doctor will make sure the baby's head, organs, and body size are developing according to plan. Usually the technician will give you your first picture of the baby from the ultrasound.

To check for birth defects that can occur when the cells of the fetus start multiplying, a procedure called amniocentesis is sometimes recommended. This test is especially important if a pregnant woman is older than thirty-five or has had genetic, developmental problems with other pregnancies. Special technicians perform this test, taking some amniotic fluid that surrounds the baby and examining it to make sure the baby will be free from difficulties, like Down's Syndrome. It is a good test to have if you need it because decisions can be made concerning family planning, or giving the baby what he or she will need before birth to be healthier after delivery.

## Hepatitis and HIV

There are two infectious diseases that everybody needs to be informed and educated about. These diseases are spread from one person to another, mostly by exposure to blood-contaminated items like injection needles or blood transfusions, and through sexual contact with someone who is infected. These two scary, serious diseases are hepatitis and HIV. Hang in there to learn the truth about HIV and hepatitis because these germs are damaging to everybody. The more you know, the better you can protect yourself and your baby.

Your healthcare professionals will probably want to check you for these diseases with lab tests; let them. People can have these diseases and not know it, so none of us can tell who is okay unless we've been tested. Every pregnant woman should be tested. She will be treated with good medicine and counseling if she needs it.

Hepatitis is a disease that damages the liver, the largest organ in your body. The liver has many important jobs, like storing vitamins until needed and changing food products in the blood to nourishment. The liver is where red blood cells, which carry oxygen from your lungs to your tissues, are stored for a baby's growth. In order for healthcare people to take good care of a pregnant woman, they test for hepatitis. Another type of hepatitis can get into your body from feces (bowel movement). Wash your hands and your children's hands after using the bathroom or diapering a child. Can you think of another disease that hurts the liver? Drinking alcohol can cause it—cirrhosis.

HIV/AIDS is a virus, a germ, that attacks the immune system in your body. You have organs and special blood cells that protect you from getting infections from germs that are picked up just by being around people. Usually people do not become sick from these germs because their immune system is healthy. HIV (Human Immunodeficiency Virus) breaks down this protective system. When HIV-positive people become susceptible to bacterial infections, like pneumonia, endocarditis (inflammation of the heart), tuberculosis, hepatitis, sexually transmitted diseases, and cancers, they are said to have AIDS (Acquired Immune Deficiency Syndrome). Sometimes HIV infected people show symptoms of the disease, and sometimes they don't feel sick or look sick for many years. Without knowing they have it, HIV-positive people can and do give the virus to others.

Protect yourself: don't let anyone's body fluids, such as semen or blood, enter your body unless it's doctor-recommended. Enjoy sexual activities without intercourse or oral sex, or use a condom and a lubricant each and every time. Don't share needles, razor blades, or anything else that comes in contact with another person's blood and semen. Get tested—breast milk also transmits the virus.

If mom is positive for the HIV virus, an unborn baby can become infected because they share the same blood supply. Newborns are at risk if mom breast feeds. The good news is even if mom is HIV-positive, there is a 60 to 90 percent chance the baby will not have HIV, and not develop AIDS. These are very good, hopeful odds. The chances of a baby getting the disease from an HIV-positive mom depend on how long she's had the infection, or if she's received medical treatment for it. The doctors can do a lot to protect and help women and babies, so get the test and know you did everything you could do and should do for you and your baby's future.

Get your lab tests done as soon as possible, grin and bear it, and find an understanding, knowledgeable person to talk to. Ask questions and express your feelings about these diseases and having to wait for the results. It is definitely better to know your body's condition now, rather than after the baby is born. Why? Because doctors can make a world of difference in a baby's health by giving a pregnant woman the right medical attention. Ask for the help and support you need at this time, and keep reading! You are being very brave, smart, and strong, by learning the facts of pregnancy, prenatal care, and all that goes with it.

By getting examinations, laboratory tests, and other prenatal care procedures, you are giving yourself an extra-special bonus. How you feel about yourself will change. You would be taking actions that are worthy of respect—the actions of a responsible, concerned mother. The good things you do will give you feelings of worthiness, self-respect, and pride. You will have much to be proud of if you take the actions that will help you stay well by getting prenatal care and drug and alcohol treatment. Think of how happy you will feel when your baby is born better than she or he could have been, because you took care of business.

Addictive behaviors like drug and alcohol use tear you down and rip families apart. Please choose to do those things that build you up, while your baby is being "built." The life force inside of you will beat stronger, happier, and more confidently. Women who feel good about what they are doing in their lives, no matter what has happened in their past, get the strength to stay away from people who give pregnant women drugs and alcohol, steer clear of dangerous situations, and keep moving in a positive direction. You will be able to ignore harmful influences when you feel you and your baby deserve better. And you do deserve good things in your life. Every mom and baby does. Nice work, mom—keep on reading!

# CHAPTER 5

# The Bottom Line on Babies, Drugs, and Alcohol

Babies are marvelous people with unbelievable capacities to make it across many obstacles to healthy growth. From a few multiplying cells to a fully developed newborn, a human being is created in nine short months. Wow! Every baby is born with a special personality and unique emotional and physical characteristics, just as you were.

Your drug and alcohol dependencies changed the real you, and directed your life's course. Substance use by mom, whether during pregnancy or while parenting, will change your baby's personality and physical condition, too.

The information in this chapter is not to be used as a club to beat yourself with, or as a way to put yourself down. You have experienced enough guilt and pain. While learning the truth about infant drug and alcohol exposure, be sweet to yourself at the times you need it most—while you are getting better and building your life back up. So don't even think about picking up the club.

By continuing to read this survival guide and preparing your-self, you can stack the deck so that that your physical and emo-tional influences upon a developing baby will be positive, healthy, and life-giving. We have come to know that depending on drugs and alcohol to live produces the opposite effect—death. Let's make sure the odds are in your favor. You do not want to gamble any longer with your baby's health, or yours, in this real-life game where the players often pay too high a price. You have already paid your dues to addiction. Your baby doesn't have to.

Knowledge is power. You will always be a strong force in your child's life but never as powerfully as when you are carrying your baby. Without the knowledge of how drugs and alcohol can hurt an infant's mental and physical growth, your addictions could get the upper hand. Addiction, we have already learned, can trick you into denial so you'll end up back where you started, or worse. Your newborn would then begin life with less healthy tis-sue, and fewer good brain and nerve cells, which a baby will need to become the terrific person she or he was meant to be.

Here is something solid for you to hold onto that no one can take away from you—knowledge. Use this information to hang onto what you want in your life to be happy. The more you know, the more your choices will be good ones in the days and years to come. So fasten your seat belt, know that you have love and good-ness in your heart, and keep reading—you're going in the right direction.

## The Basic Facts About Alcohol, Drugs, and a Baby in the Womb

This general information comes from medical professionals, public health people, child development specialists, and others who have cared for substance-exposed babies. They have studied infant health problems and written about what they've learned in order to teach all of us how to help affected newborns, their mothers, and their families.

We know that any kind of drug or type of alcohol is harmful to the minds and bodies of adults, children, and babies. Anything that gets you high, intoxicated, or under the influence, can lead to a physical and psychological dependency upon addictive chemicals. When drug and alcohol use is stopped (abstinence), mild to severe withdrawal symptoms can be experienced by babies, as well as by adults, if substances have been inside their bodies. The single most important reason alcohol and drug use is so serious is that these chemicals affect the central nervous system. This system consists of your brain and spinal cord.

The brain is the control center of your body that translates and communicates important information to body parts, for example, through the spinal cord to the muscles in your arms and hands. This relay of information allows you to think, reach, flex for strength, and pick up something or someone safely, like a baby.

The brain allows us to think, feel emotions, learn language, and understand what we hear, see, smell, taste, and touch. It enables us to respond to what is happening around us. Your brain is in charge of almost everything you do, like hearing a baby cry, remembering that it's time to feed the baby, and enjoying the feeling of holding an infant in your arms.

All types of alcohol and drugs mix with the good chemicals and their receptors that are already in your brain, and a reaction happens. That's why people feel high or low while under the influence of drugs and alcohol. People experience physical effects, too, like stumbling around or, while driving, not reacting fast enough to hit the brakes and avoid another car. Were children in the car with a driver who was loaded? That's something worth thinking about.

The only time your baby can develop enough brain cells for thinking and learning good behavior is prenatally (when babies are growing in their mothers' wombs) and during the first few months after birth. After this time, a human brain cannot increase the number of cells it needs to work well. What mom eats, drinks, smokes, shoots up, or snorts while pregnant can cause malnutrition; the developing baby would not get the blood, oxygen, and food needed to grow brain and nerve cells. Since a baby's brain develops completely during the first few months of life, it's really important that newborns have someone to feed them the right kind and the right amount of formula or breast milk at the right time. Someone like you.

The other major part of the central nervous system is the spinal cord. Like roots growing from the trunk of a tree, the spinal cord's nerves go from the brain to every area of our bodies. These nerve fibers are like a two-way street. For example, information goes from the brain to our feet, telling them to walk. Information also goes from our feet to the brain, when, for instance, we step on a thorn. Someone who steps on a thorn doesn't have to think, "Gee, do I have something stuck in my foot?" We know right away, and respond in a flash to the pain by lifting our foot, looking for the thorn, and maybe saying a few coarse words, without even thinking about it. We react immediately. These reflexes, which rely on the brain to explain the sensation of pain, and the spinal cord nerves that relay this information, are necessary for us to survive as we move around in the world, or in the womb.

Many substance-abusing pregnant women believe that if their baby is born a little jittery and shaky or sleepy with dull, glassy eyes, that the child will be all right, that it's not a big deal. Women who have used substances while pregnant with other children often feel this way. They see that their kids have two arms and two legs, and assume that any problems from drug and alcohol exposure aren't really serious because the children will grow out of it. But this is not the truth of the situation.

If a newborn is trembling and jittery, the baby's nervous system has been harmed. Jerky movements are the muscles and nerve fibers reacting unpredictably, which the baby cannot control. A baby who can't stop moving around or is shivering and trembling, will not be able to stay calm enough to eat, sleep, respond, or grow normally. A baby can also be drowsy, unalert, and sleep so much that he or she must be awakened to eat. This is a big deal.

Infants whose nervous systems have either been overstimulated or depressed from exposure to drugs and alcohol, will have trouble. Often they cannot enjoy a mother's smile, the sounds around them, bright sunlight, the feeling of their blankets, or a bunch of admiring people. Their brains and nerves can't handle all this activity and information that's coming at them. This is really important because when babies feel stressed or are unable to stay alert, they don't have those interested eyes or joyful smiles that moms and others look for when they interact with a child. It becomes harder for both mother and baby to bond, to share special moments, to get to know each other's face and emotions. It's hard to get as close to each other as they want to be and need to be.

Nature designed the greatest survival tool for babies—the attachment that happens between a mother/caretaker and a child. Drug and alcohol exposure gets in the way of this natural, enjoyable bonding experience. Bonding is really important for mothers, too. Moms yearn for it and expect it. If mom isn't clean and sober, her emotional and physical presence is different and could prevent her from communicating and bonding with her baby in a real, natural, genuine manner. Don't let alcohol and drugs take nature's gift of bonding away from you and your baby.

Almost all chemically dependent people use more than one substance—like tobacco, alcohol, and various prescription and illegal drugs—at the same time. It is important for women to know that using more than one substance during your baby's development will increase the chances of problems and the seriousness of those problems. Multiple chemicals in a woman's body become mixed up and interact in her brain and in her womb so it is hard for medical people to know in what way a baby will be affected.

Secondary chemicals are added to drugs when they are manufactured. Tobacco, for example, is treated with additives while being processed. Because many substance abusers use illegal drugs, they can never be sure of the quality, or how much of the drug, or what kind of toxic additive they are putting into their bodies. Illegal drug and narcotic manufacturers want to dilute the drug to increase their profit. It's no secret that dealers get money from making and selling drugs. They are probably not concerned with sanitary, germ-free conditions, toxic additives, or your health when the substances are made. These facts increase the dangers of drug and alcohol use, especially since a growing baby will receive these additives, too.

Finally, the way drugs and alcohol are taken into your body determines if they hit your central nervous system (brain and spinal cord) in five seconds or fifteen minutes. How chemically dependent people use their drugs increases the harmful effects. For example, smoking and injecting causes drugs to get to your brain faster than inhaling substances through the nose or taking them orally. The faster you become intoxicated, the more your brain and body has to deal with all the chemicals in drugs and alcohol.

Some drug use, like smoking cocaine or inhalants, produces a temporary high. Then addicts quickly want to use again. So they smoke and inhale more. Although injecting is a fast way to get drugs in your body, chemicals like heroin, pills (barbiturates, tranquilizers, and sedatives), and hallucinogens, also have long-lasting effects, up to twenty-four hours. The longer you've used, the less your body will be able to fight these chemicals and eliminate them from your body.

Some drugs stay in your body a long time. PCP and marijuana remain in your body a lot longer because the body stores these substances in the fat cells. Your body puts alcohol and other drugs into the fluids of cells, and the watery fluids travel out more quickly, but are no less damaging. All drugs, including alcohol, are truly body- and mind-altering chemicals.

We've learned that the fluid around the baby and mom's flow of blood nourishes a baby, allowing him or her to grow. When a pregnant woman uses or drinks, alcohol and all types of drugs are active inside the placenta, floating in the amniotic fluid, umbilical cord, and bloodstream. A fetus' and baby's organs are not well developed and cannot excrete or get rid of chemicals as an adult's body can. This means a baby is exposed to the substances longer because they are in the baby's organs, cells, and surrounding fluids. During their prenatal development, babies can be thought of as being like little sponges, especially when drugs and alcohol are present.

All pregnant women need to know that their baby's health depends on many factors in addition to being alcohol- and drug-free. Women can have a lot of control over things that will improve the health of developing babies, such as: eating habits (good nutrition), general state of health (no infections or diseases), sleeping habits (getting enough uninterrupted rest), obtaining good prenatal care (early and often), living conditions (stable housing that is clean with all necessities like water and power), and domestic peace and relaxation (no battering or emotional abuse). Some health areas cannot be changed, and a woman has little control over her family's genetic characteristics (inherited weaknesses in certain physical areas), some types of mental illness, and if she has been abused in childhood.

Let's give your addictions a run for your money. Three things are certain:

- I believe in the scientific law of cause and effect. If a mother-to-be drinks alcohol or uses drugs, these substances are the cause and somewhere, somehow, there will be an effect.

- No one can predict with certainty what kind of problems will occur in a growing baby when chemicals are in a mother's body.

- Frequent, early prenatal care will improve a baby's health, even if mom drank or used during pregnancy.

It needs to be known—the disease of drug addiction and alcoholism can be fatal to infants as well as adults. How can we be sure? Because it's happened.

## Effects of Drugs and Alcohol on Babies

Some general facts have been proven time and time again. Remember—no beating yourself up while you're learning. Let's go through some effects here, because whether "your thing" is alcohol, cocaine, methamphetamine, PCP, pills (uppers or downers, by prescription or illegally manufactured), heroin, hallucinogens, or marijuana, infant bodies are affected in similar ways.

Drugs and alcohol can cause children to be born smaller (growth retardation), earlier (premature), and to weigh less (low birth weight). Babies born smaller than they should be cannot keep their body temperature stable as the air changes around them, and are more susceptible to sweating and illness, like respiratory and lung infections.

Small babies have smaller heads, and therefore, smaller brains than full-term, normal growth and weight babies. The head and the brain cannot grow enough to catch up after the baby has been born. These kids can have trouble learning, listening, paying attention, speaking—it all starts in the brain. Since chemicals affect the spinal cord as well, drug- and alcohol-exposed children usually have poor physical coordination. This is especially harsh for babies, who may not be able to move their jaw, mouth, and throat properly to suck a bottle or breast and then swallow. They have trouble eating, sleeping, and it becomes difficult for them to gain weight.

Babies affected by alcohol and drugs are often unhappy, irritable, and difficult to calm down or to wake up. They need more holding, soothing, feeding, changing, and the right kind of attention from their caretakers. Sometimes it becomes a pain, rather than a pleasure, to take care of their needs. A distressed infant adds a ton of stress on those people, like mothers, who have to fulfill a baby's normal demands, and probably aren't getting enough sleep themselves.

People who take care of babies are human and can become tired and frustrated. Sometimes this stress leads to the possibility of neglect or abuse of these special babies who need all the help and love they can get. Mothers and babies have a rough time if drugs and alcohol are in the family picture.

## Alcohol and Depressants

Alcohol works just like a drug in your brain and body. It is a depressant, which means it decreases your mental and physical ability to function. Other depressant drugs come in pill form, for example, tranquilizers (Valium, Halcion, Xanax) and sedatives (barbiturates, methaqualone). Since the physical and mental effects of alcohol and other depressant drugs are similar in babies and adults, let's talk about them together.

Alcohol is a useful chemical, outside your body. Remember how a nurse cleans your skin with an alcohol swab before giving you a shot or putting a bandage on a cut? Alcohol kills fast growing cells like bacteria that would make you sick if they got into your blood.

What is a fetus? A bunch of very fast growing cells. Alcohol destroys and damages those cells. You've read that an infant's first red blood cells are made in mom's liver, which is where alcohol is mostly processed by the body. There is no way to tell if one alcoholic drink, or five drinks, is safe for a woman to have if she's pregnant. A can of beer has the same amount of alcohol as a glass of wine or a shot of whiskey, so any alcoholic beverage can cause problems. Honestly, there isn't any type of alcohol, or amount of beer, wine, or liquor that can be consumed safely by a pregnant woman.

What alcohol and depressant drug use can do to a growing baby is really important to know. Damage from alcohol and downers has been found in many children to be permanent, no matter what kind or how much help mothers, doctors, and infant specialists give. Babies, inside or outside of the womb, can go through withdrawal, overdose, seizures, and have reductions in heart rate, breathing, movement, blood pressure, and nerve and brain activity, just like adults.

Many women are offered tranquilizers and sedatives by relatives, friends, or perhaps by doctors or therapists. If you are pregnant, you need to know that these pills are strong medicine, highly concentrated, that can cause birth defects. Don't take any pills while pregnant, even over-the-counter medications like aspirin, until you talk to your OB healthcare doctor or nurse first.

Some women need medication and a doctor's close supervision for mental illness. If you're not one of them, don't let anyone, even your own mother, talk you into taking a pill to relax or sleep, or any other drug. You will not feel better. The chemical will be passed from your body into your baby, and would show on a laboratory test.

During prenatal development, alcohol exposure can cause mental retardation and lowered intelligence, abnormal features of the face, and poorly developed ears and other structures. A baby's growth can be stunted; that is, staying too small as a child and as an adult. Babies with these problems have fetal alcohol syndrome (FAS) or fetal alcohol effect (FAE), and will not be able to take care of themselves as adults because they can't learn how.

Not drinking alcohol after the second trimester has been found to decrease the likelihood of FAS. But who can tell which babies will end up with FAE learning disabilities, FAS mental retardation, or which ones might escape the most damaging effects of alcohol? The reality is: as soon as you're pregnant the only course to take is to stop drinking. If you're still having a drink or two, start screaming and calling for help. Abstaining from alcohol and downers will definitely benefit your child's natural growth and thinking ability. The life you save may be your baby's.

## *Stimulants*

Cocaine and amphetamine or methamphetamine are almost exactly alike in the way they operate as chemicals in the body. The form a drug comes in doesn't matter, whether it's smokable, inhalable, crystallized, made into a pill, or whatever. These chemicals work the same way in your brain and body. These drugs are uppers or stimulants to your central nervous system. We don't call amphetamine "speed" for nothing!

The most common effects of these stimulant drugs in babies are prematurity (from pre-term contractions of mom's stimulated uterus), overall retarded development, and problems in the way a baby's organs and tissues are formed from mom's decreased blood flow. The workings of the brain and spinal cord are injured, putting babies at risk for feeding, movement, and other problems, some of which can be improved given the right help and loving parenting techniques. Later in life, a drug- and alcohol-exposed child frequently has difficulty with good behavior, schoolwork, and maintaining an attention span that's appropriate to the child's age.

It's very sad that infants who are born to drug- and alcohol-dependent mothers are at higher risk—five to ten times higher, for sudden infant death syndrome (SIDS) than babies who have not been exposed. Crib death, or SIDS, usually occurs between the ages of three weeks and seven months. You will learn special techniques in chapter 7 that show you how to position and comfort your baby. Then you'll both feel better and less fearful. Hang in there and keep reading, because you are doing a remarkable job!

## *Narcotics*

Many prescription drugs contain opiates, which means these medicines are narcotics. Don't be fooled—Tylenol No. 3 and No. 4,

Robitussin AC, and Cheracol cough syrups all contain codeine. Other narcotics include Dilaudid, Percodan, and Darvon and they are as highly addictive as heroin.

Opiate addiction from heroin, codeine, morphine, and other narcotics gets very complicated, as every addict knows. Women addicted to these drugs frequently suffer from inflammation of their veins (thrombophlebitis) and heart (endocarditis), and are at high risk of being infected with hepatitis and HIV, especially if they are injection drug users. It is vital to use condoms every time you have sex; don't share needles, ever; keep up with healthcare visits; and, if you haven't already, think about a methadone maintenance program.

Infants exposed to heroin and other narcotics will go through withdrawal symptoms, some severe, some less traumatic. The symptoms sometimes take up to ten days to be seen in a baby, coming and going and maybe coming back again. Narcotic-affected newborns need lots of medical supervision, attention, and often medication to calm them during withdrawal. They are usually hard to soothe and less alert, with tremors, stiffness, and decreased vision. As with almost all drug and alcohol use, opiate-exposed newborns frequently show weight and growth retardation unless mom gets early prenatal care (but you knew that, right?) and methadone.

The best reason for a narcotic-addicted woman to get methadone the minute she knows she's pregnant is that the doctors and nurses cannot handle heroin and other drug complications in a newborn as well as they can manage methadone effects in a baby. The amount of methadone can be monitored in the baby because it can be monitored in mom. If the choice is between continued illicit drug use and other risky behavior or taking methadone, choose methadone. Detoxing yourself from narcotics while pregnant is traumatic for your brain and body, and puts the baby in withdrawal, too.

Methadone is recommended for pregnant opiate addicts to decrease spontaneous abortion, health problems in the baby, and contracting infectious diseases from risky activities. Methadone maintenance early and throughout pregnancy was found to help babies grow longer in mom's uterus, have better weight at delivery time, and have better growth because mom's nutrition and lifestyle improved. With proper assistance, these children often catch up in development by six months of age.

If you are opiate addicted, methadone is a loving, responsible, humane thing to do for yourself and for your baby. This substance decreases physical and emotional suffering, and enables you to live a more normal life, show up for prenatal care, stay away from active users, and not have to chase after or hustle your drugs. What a relief!

## *Hallucinogens*

Using PCP (phencyclidine) or taking prescription drugs that are hypnotics is particularly dangerous because of their effects on the central nervous system. This type of drug use causes sensory deprivation, like extreme numbness, and users don't feel the pain or discomfort they should from an injury. And, they get injured a lot from being unable to recognize danger while under the influence. People who use PCP and other drugs have suffered amnesia, convulsions, and coma. Infants prenatally exposed to PCP and pills are often found to have unique, unpredictable problems in the way their nervous systems work. These little ones have extreme, quickly changing moods that they can't control; they are easily startled, upset, and generally shook up for a long time. Fortunately, these children usually do not have retarded structural growth prenatally or low birth weight.

Nerve damage from PCP and other drugs is serious and can produce big behavioral problems in children as they grow older. An exposed child who cannot regulate (keep a lid on) emotions has trouble controlling his or her temper and stopping misbehavior. Some PCP-exposed children cannot understand right from wrong. By not being aware of the consequences of their actions, these affected children become confused, angry adolescents and adults who feel insecure and aggressive. They are at risk for an unhappy life, in their homes and in society. Be an angel, and stay away from the dust.

One doesn't have to be a genius to know that hallucinogenic drugs can cause injury to the brain, spinal cord, and bodies of babies and adults. Hallucinogens deeply change the way people comprehend what they hear, see, taste, smell, and touch. What if an addict hears the sound of a vacuum cleaner, believes it to be someone drilling into his or her brain, and is found wandering the streets five days later? You get the idea, and it's a true story. Whether it is made by man (LSD, MDMA, MDA, XTC, mescaline) or nature (psilocybin "magic mushrooms," mescaline "peyote," DMT "businessman's special"), the drug effect from these chemicals is intense and can last up to twelve hours or days.

Because of these drugs' strong action on the brain and emotions, men and women experience hallucinations, delusions, panic, paranoia, depression, and maybe colorful visions. People don't know ahead of time if their unreal trip will be fun or even if they will return from it. The drug effects are real, truly harmful, and too dangerous for both users and everyone around them.

People who take hallucinogenic drugs, cocaine, PCP, alcohol, and methamphetamine are vulnerable to psychosis as well. This serious symptom is a mental disturbance that causes the user to lose contact with reality and tears apart one's self-identity. Psychosis causes people to not know who they are or believe they are someone else, like Jesus Christ or Madonna. While in a psychotic state, addicts and alcoholics have crazy ideas or no idea about what they're doing or why they're doing it. They can feel deathly depressed or superhumanly powerful. This experience is painful and frightening. People need to be hospitalized for psychosis brought on by addictive chemicals. Pick up a travel magazine about Hawaii, bake some cookies, or take a walk, because any trip is better for you and your baby than those that are drug induced.

## Marijuana

Many substance-abusing women feel marijuana isn't as harmful to use as other drugs while they are pregnant. It grows out of the ground (but so does cocaine), it's like an herb, everybody smokes it, and so on. But the facts are in 'and they're clear. The chemical in marijuana that gets you high stays in your body, and in your baby, a long time. Marijuana-exposed babies typically have low birth weight, withdrawal symptoms (believe it), respiratory illnesses, and are also at risk for heart problems and crib death. If you are a mother or a mother-to-be, don't pick up that joint or pipe. No matter who is smoking it, you don't have to, my friend.

## Cigarettes

Gotta talk about it—smoking cigarettes. We learned that tobacco contains many harmful chemicals besides the nicotine that gets people addicted to smoking. Smokers experience more pregnancy complications and still births. Babies whose mothers have smoked during pregnancy had lower birth weights than mothers who didn't smoke. Newborns tend to have respiratory illnesses (bronchitis, asthma, pneumonia), ear infections, and are at risk for SIDS. Secondary smoke from a cigarette causes fluid to build up in children's small lungs and tiny ear canals. For you, the smoker, here's the latest: smoking has made cancer the number one killer of American women. Perhaps now, or in the future, you will have the desire to quit smoking, and can ask for help and receive loving support to stop.

A wonderful writer wrote the following poem to help us all on our journey toward health and happiness.

What lies behind us
and what lies before us
are tiny matters compared to
what lies within us.

Ralph Waldo Emerson

# CHAPTER 6

# Ready or Not,
# the Baby's Comin'

Within weeks or months your baby will be born. Wherever you are starting in terms of your recovery from chemical dependency, this chapter will tell you how to have the best possible delivery experience. Learning how to take care of yourself, getting the services you need, and understanding hospital procedures will help you cope with today, and have a better tomorrow.

We know that getting good, frequent prenatal care, and showing up for drug and alcohol treatment and recovery meetings is necessary to prepare your mind and your body for a life worth living—healthy and free from alcohol and drug use. These are the first steps toward having what you want: life, love, and the freedom to pursue happiness with your children. Now, preparing for the baby's arrival is the next step, and it begins with learning what you need to do, and doing it. You're on top of it, so keep reading!

These suggestions are important because they will benefit you, your baby, and your family. Following through in getting these needs met will also show others you have taken responsible action toward insuring your baby's welfare. The recommendations explained below are not being pulled out of a hat. These are a few of the things that healthcare professionals, family members, hospital social service people, and children's services workers look for if problems related to substance abuse arise. Mothers and others need to make sure a baby will be cared for and safe. If you haven't already started your preparations, please know that taking care of business now will help your baby and can save you from an enormous amount of heartache later. So let's go to it, and no cheating.

## Home Environment

A parent must make sure they have a clean and safe home for a baby. This home environment, inside and outside, should be free of hazards, like roaches, rodents (rats), or stray animals; holes in the wall or ground; dirty carpets; or unsafe, exposed wiring of refrigerators and other electrical appliances. Check the operation of your room heater and stove. Pull out all poisonous, toxic items (cleaning solutions, bleach, bug spray, car oil, and so on) and put them on a high shelf. Hopefully by now, the addictive poisons of alcohol and drugs are not in the place where you live. Have the baby's clothes, bedding, diapers, formula, and other baby articles washed, organized, and covered with a clean cloth or sheet.

All you need in terms of the big stuff is a crib, a car seat, and a front pack or sling made of strong reinforced fabric with which to carry your baby securely on your chest. Like kangaroo babies who grow strong in mom's pouch, human babies need to be close to their mothers. For infants to feel secure, they need to hear mom's voice and heartbeat, and enjoy her warmth and smell. For newborns at risk this is the best way to carry and comfort babies when you stand or walk until they are about four months of age, or older if your baby was born prematurely. When bending over or getting on a bus, be sure to support the baby's head and bend at the knees, not from the back. A sling or front pack is much better for new babies than the hard plastic carrier seats where the baby's position is limited and mother's body is far away. You can use a stroller later on for your baby's safety and for your convenience.

Motherhood is probably the biggest job a woman will ever have. It takes courage to let relatives and other people know you are serious about having a calm and safe place for your baby, and for your recovery from alcoholism and drug addiction. Think of how protective a lioness would be with her cubs. If you share a home with others, ask them to smoke outside and keep booze and drugs out of there. Don't let your house become Grand Central Station, with people running in and out.

If you live in an area with community unrest or gang violence, make sure you have curtains on the windows and adequate locks on the doors, and that people are not hanging around your house or apartment. A kind, concerned call or letter to the property manager or landlord asking for their assistance might help. Keep track of the things you have tried to improve in your home environment by writing them down.

A lot of women left home while they were teenagers, and never learned the basics about cleaning and organizing a home. Good housekeeping is a concrete way to show how much you care for your children, and how concerned you are about protecting your newborn from outside influences, like germs, noise, cold temperatures, and bad air. If you clean your home by throwing everything in a closet, ask a relative or a friend to show you the best, easiest way to do housework. The only people who should feel ashamed are those who don't ask for help and advice when they need it in order to learn a better way to do things. Remember— you don't need a penthouse, new furniture, or much money to make a safe, comfortable nest for your baby and a home you can feel good about.

## Getting Assistance

If you do not have the baby articles or household items you need, now's the time to reach out. Become a detective to locate churches, secondhand stores, and social service organizations in your town that can give you or lend you what you need. Friends and neighbors might have things that their children have outgrown. Tell them you are trying to change your life (if you're reading this guide, you are) by following directions for recovery, and that you need a little help to prepare for the baby's arrival.

If a prenatal care nurse has not suggested it, ask to talk to the hospital or OB clinic social worker who can tell you where to go for assistance in getting what you need for your baby. Make a list, and take it with you. Healthcare social workers also know where to refer you for emergency food, housing, childcare, and perhaps transportation assistance. This is a big part of their job—to help families access social services and ongoing healthcare in the community.

If you do not have a source of income or someone providing for your needs that doesn't have a string attached, you should obtain some aid so you can provide for the baby. The hospital social worker can tell you where to go and what you'll need to take with you to apply for Medi-Cal or Medicaid, Aid to Families with Dependent Children (AFDC) and Women's, Infant's, and Children's Nutrition Program (WIC) at the Department of Public Social Services. This agency will need to see your identification, a verification of pregnancy (you can get this from your OB nurse), and other papers to sign you up.

Again, the only women who should feel crummy about getting county aid entitlement are those who need this help for their families and *don't* apply for it, or those who don't need assistance and are getting it! People who are still boozing and using are typically not able to make it to the service agencies they need to contact. Don't be one of them. Take a good book to read, a snack to eat, some (or maybe a lot of) patience, and the papers you'll need to get these benefits with a minimum of hassle. The more you know, the better prepared you'll be and the less stressed you'll become. If you don't feel stressed, it will be easier to stay clean and sober as you go through the process of obtaining county and community services.

If you are drug- and alcohol-free while obtaining services for your family, you will definitely have a better chance of succeeding in these tasks with the least amount of problems. If your primary desire is to have a healthy baby and a happy home, getting busy and preparing for an infant's arrival is the best way to meet this goal. By asking for help, following through, and recovering from your addictions, you can end up where you want to be—with your baby, safe at home.

## Why Parenting Classes?

Babies do not come with instruction booklets. We know that our parents didn't get a "how-to" manual when we were born that taught them how to take care of us. No offense to your parents, but much has been discovered in the past ten years about new, proven parenting techniques. Every parent can learn more about kids with up-to-date information that is especially important when children have been affected by drug and alcohol addiction in their family.

*Kids learn what to do and how to behave because their mother knew how to teach them.* Knowing the most useful ways to communicate with and discipline children, and what babies should be doing as they grow, means less frustration and worry for mom and is help-ful for kids. You are probably a pretty exciting person, so grab onto some new, exciting parenting skills.

Drug- and alcohol-dependent people have often been out of school or away from learning situations for a long time. Were you ever told you were stupid, or not good in school? If you were, don't believe it, and prove them wrong. You're on the ball if you participate in a prenatal or parenting class. Anyone can be a good listener and everyone should ask a lot of questions when learning something new.

Continuing your education in this way is great for you, and will be super for your baby. If your drug and alcohol treatment program does not have prenatal or parenting classes, ask your OB nurse or hospital social worker for a referral to one that's afford-able or free, and near your home. Many healthcare facilities have parenting classes, as well as community and private organizations that work with children. Ask and you shall receive the most bene-ficial skills on caring for your baby and dealing with your kids. By learning all you can about good parenting, you will know what to do, and will do it better, than someone who hasn't taken the time to attend a parenting or prenatal education class.

The better prepared you are, the more at ease you will be with your baby. Babies are sensitive to mother's emotions. When they sense that mom is fearful, worried, angry, or spaced-out, infants can feel nervous and begin to cry. Learn the best tools to feel less afraid and to become more confident in handling your helpless, possibly fragile newborn. Obtaining the services you need, and knowing what you're doing in order to help your baby are great ways to relieve stress!

# Dealing with Fear

Labor and delivery are pretty stressful times for many people— mom, doctors, nurses, the family, and the baby. Some drug- and alcohol-dependent pregnant women don't make it to the hospital because of their fear of new experiences, or fear that their substance use may be discovered. Their babies are born at home in the toilet, in an ambulance, a dope house, or worse. No one would want to stop her baby from getting the best medical care, even if a baby is going to be placed for adoption. Yet it happens. Drugs and alcohol can be more powerful than a mother's good intentions, and can stop her from doing the right thing for a baby at risk. Don't let addictions keep you from the hospital. It's not worth it, in the short-term or in the long run, and the newborn will suffer.

If you have been receiving prenatal care, you will at least feel okay about going to the hospital. It will be easier to work with the doctors and nurses because you have a relationship with them already. Ask someone in the prenatal care clinic to give you a tour of the OB ward, labor and delivery rooms, and nurseries, so you can become familiar with where you and your baby will be in the hospital come delivery time.

For most alcoholics and drug addicts, it's become hard to trust other people, to get along with them, and to relate to others effectively. Earlier in life, it was easy to feel left out, and ongoing addictive behaviors kept individuals feeling alone and troubled in their casual, as well as their close, intimate relationships. When faced with strangers in a hospital, a baby's impending birth, and feelings of fear and guilt, a substance-abusing woman may want to respond defensively to other people. The shame of chemical dependency makes reality and honesty difficult to deal with. Being angry, blaming and hating caregivers, denying that problems exist, or withdrawing emotionally are some ways women express their pain, fear, and frustration.

Anger can be a very useful, positive emotion for an addicted mother, if handled in the right way. If she is angry at what she did or didn't do, this can be the beginning of truthfulness, an opening up, and a motivation for changing her life. The answer to feelings of anger and pain is the same for chemically dependent women as it is for doctors, nurses, social workers, or anyone; it's okay to feel angry at situations we find ourselves in. It's okay to let pain out, to cry and feel despair or sorrow when we feel bad about ourselves, or feel bad for another, like a child. What's not okay for anyone to do is threaten, attack, or punish other people with words or actions because of how we feel. And what most people really feel is fear.

Alcohol- and drug-dependent women are afraid for themselves, their baby, and their family when their abuse of substances is exposed. Chemical dependency is recognized most often from physical symptoms seen in mom or baby; laboratory tests of mom, baby, or both; mom's behavior; or her honesty about her substance use.

Doctors, nurses, and other hospital personnel also experience a lot of feelings. Delivery of an infant is an emotionally charged situation for almost everyone, particularly when the health of patients has been influenced by drugs and alcohol. All persons involved need to make sure their fear or anger does not allow them to act in ways that hurt, rather than help.

You can handle your painful emotions in a way that will not be harmful to you or others during your hospital stay. Understanding that anger, fear, and shame are likely to surface and are normal feelings for anyone in this situation can help you stay in control. Try not to scare yourself with horrible, terrorizing thoughts about what could happen next. No one has a crystal ball that can see your future. By focusing on the worst possible outcome or jumping to negative conclusions, you are setting yourself up to react that way—really negatively.

Don't let what is going on around you trigger your worst behavior. It could come back to haunt you. Remembering what the enemy is (and it isn't a person, not even you) might help. Losing your cool, verbally or physically attacking someone, or refusing to talk to healthcare personnel, will not get you where you want to be. Leaving the hospital without being medically discharged, or running away before problems can be explained or settled could be considered abandonment of the baby.

*Don't let this happen to you. You and your baby are worth saving!*

Being kind to yourself during the stress of labor, delivery, and afterwards is a wonderful thing for a chemically dependent woman to do for herself. Saying nice words to yourself, silently or aloud, imagining someone you love hugging you, or thinking of scenes that inspire you, like a golden sunset, will help you stay calm, patient, and in a better place to handle any problems that might come up.

Express how you feel to the people around you, without acting on how you feel. This means you can be honest with your feelings, telling hospital caregivers or others that you feel hurt, sad, upset, or whatever, but don't act out your pain or frustration by yelling, cursing, throwing things, ignoring people, or splitting. The disease of addiction is used to having its way with you and helping you fail. Don't let it. Take the pressure off by talking about it, not by behaving emotionally, mentally, or physically out of control.

Keeping yourself together and letting other people help you will move you closer to your goal of having a healthier family. Knowing you need to take care of yourself, emotionally and physically, so you can be there for your children, is a great attitude to have. Repeating phrases to yourself like "I'm going to hang in there, no matter what," "I'm going to have a baby who needs me," and "I'm going to be all right,"will help a fearful woman through the stress of delivery and postpartum blues, even when she is feeling love, guilt, relief, and hate, all at the same time. Being cooperative, concerned about your own health and the baby's condition, and willing to talk about problems and work through difficulties are the best ways to cope with tough situations brought about by drugs and alcohol.

# What Happens Before and After Delivery

Your body is special, and most women will agree that every childbirth is different. Labor and delivery without mom or baby in life-threatening distress is the goal. It's nice to know that you can help yourself along this uncomfortable, painful, yet fantastic experience by listening to your body and to your feelings. How you feel about yourself, your pregnancy, and your life will affect your labor. If a woman feels tense, depressed, or angry, her labor signals may be slowed and uncertain. Calm, positive emotions can speed up contractions and other normal labor signs. Some women will feel cramping on and off or false labor, and will need to rest and walk, while others will have a natural burst of energy to clean, organize, and "nest."

As your body prepares for labor, contractions felt throughout pregnancy become stronger as your uterus tightens and releases, and your cervix softens for the birth. One of the first signs is the cervix letting go of its mucus plug, called the "bloody show," allowing the opening to stretch. As your body prepares for the baby to move down, you may have diarrhea and have to urinate often to make more room. The bag of waters breaks as the baby gets into birthing position and his or her head presses against the uterus' protective membranes, releasing clear or milky amniotic fluid. If you see any brown or green stuff in the fluids or on your underwear, it could be meconium from the baby's bowels. See your doctor immediately because this could mean trouble for the baby. Most OB personnel want women to come for a checkup anyway when their water bag breaks. Some women never have a bloody show; some have slow leaking, while others feel the rush of waters breaking. Relax, mommy, but pay attention to your beginning labor signs so you can tell the nurses and the doctor what has happened. Then they will have a better idea of how you and your baby are doing. Are you clean and sober? Wonderful!

We learned that the amniotic fluid which surrounds the baby in the womb keeps her or him healthy and comfortable. After your bag of waters breaks, you need to protect your birth canal and the baby from infection. Don't put anything in your vagina—no bathing, and no last minute lovemaking, either! Drink lots of water and juices.

Crampy labor contractions frequently begin at night when women are relaxed or sleeping. Labor has three stages:

- The uterus contracts, pulling the cervical muscles up and opening (dilating) the muscles down below around the birth canal

- Pushing the baby through the birth canal

- Expelling the placenta (afterbirth) out of your body

There are many simple tools you can use to make delivery easier since you are going to be a mother soon. Find ways to relax—breathing deeply, singing to yourself, having good thoughts, talking to people who reassure you and support you, holding a favorite photograph, or hugging a blanket from home. Accepting that you are in labor and mentally focusing on the baby coming out will help while your body's under stress. Your doctor will suggest medical interventions if you need them. Loosen up, crack a smile, or cry your heart out. Express your feelings while you follow instructions from your nurse and doctor. Ask for help when you need it. Remember that every woman's labor and delivery is different, and healthcare professionals can give you some helpful tips they have learned, probably from other women in your same position! Good luck. I know you can do it, and do it well.

Following the baby's vaginal or cesarean birth, the doctors and nurses examine the child, checking temperature, breathing, heartbeat, reflexes, and appearance. The newborn will be weighed, measured, and given medicine to prevent infection. Infants are watched closely the next twenty-four hours to see how they are doing in the outside world. The healthcare professionals will take care of you, too.

The baby's medical condition will determine which nursery she or he will be placed in. Many hospitals have a regular nursery, a nursery for premature or troubled infants, and a neonatal (meaning the first weeks after birth) intensive care nursery for very sick babies. Babies can be full-term but still have low birth weight or they can be born prematurely (earlier than thirty-seven weeks). They may be smaller than would be expected for a baby at that stage of development, or a specific part of the body might have failed to grow to full-size or have trouble functioning the way it should.

You deserve to know why baby doctors (pediatricians) become concerned and are very careful in how they treat babies, especially low birth weight infants. Doctors have found that low birth weight infants are five times more likely not to make it past their first birthday than normal weight newborns. At times like this, you need to trust and believe that the medical professionals will care for and look after your baby with the best knowledge and healthcare equipment they have. You can assist the doctors and nurses in helping your baby by being available, cooperative, and truthful when asked questions or given information.

Both mother and baby may or may not experience physical symptoms or apparent medical problems related to substance abuse. Common withdrawal symptoms in newborns include mild, moderate, or severe body tremors and difficulties in sleeping, eating, waking, moving, and interacting with caregivers. High risk signs from drug and alcohol exposure can be vomiting, diarrhea, sleeping less than two hours at a time, poor sucking and feeding, high pitched crying, unresponsiveness, sluggishness, structural or reflex problems, and the necessity of medications to ease withdrawal symptoms.

A baby may need a heart monitor, IV feedings, or other treatments to improve his or her health and track progress in the nursery. If your infant needs extra-special care, you can ask the nurses to explain the procedures and the equipment that you are seeing in the nursery. *There are no dumb questions where your baby is concerned.* Having an understanding of why certain treatments are needed will help you make good decisions, be less frightened of the equipment, and feel more confident in holding your newborn.

Babies and mothers may have negative drug and alcohol laboratory screens and some withdrawal symptoms. Sometimes, either mom or baby, or both, may have a positive drug and alcohol test with few physical signs. Everyone is different and the way each person's body functions (including your baby's) is unique. Try to keep an open mind, because you can handle problems, one at a time. Remember that hospital personnel are not trying to cause you trouble, but are concerned with the health and medical conditions of their patients, like you and your baby.

## Child Protective Services

If a new mother or a newborn is suspected of having problems related to drug and alcohol use, hospital personnel are obligated to talk to the mother, perhaps the father, or family members if mom is underage. A qualified doctor, nurse, or hospital social worker may visit you in your room to explain the problems they are seeing, from physical and mental conditions to lab test results.

Healthcare personnel need to talk to you about your life and lifestyle because they need to know what substances, how often, and how much has been used during pregnancy in order for them to properly treat your baby and give excellent medical care; and they need to learn why these difficulties in babies and moms exist, from asking about family and living situations to checking parenting skills and mom's ability to manage a high risk newborn.

Hospital personnel become deeply involved because they are in the business of helping people get healthy and stay that way. In addition, healthcare organizations are required by law to notify a state agency if anyone they see is at risk for abuse or neglect. People who are at risk of being injured are women in abusive relationships, elderly or disabled persons, and minors (children). Individuals who cannot care for themselves and could be hurt or neglected by others may need assistance from a social service agency so no further harm will come to them.

Healthcare personnel, as well as government agency workers, do not want to interfere with an individual's or a family's right to privacy unless it is absolutely necessary for someone's safety and survival. Many adults and children have been abused and neglected by their caretakers. There are a lot of very sick, irresponsible, violent people out there, and laws are needed to try to stop the abuse. By 1965, all fifty states had passed laws that said doctors and other healthcare workers must notify an agency if they have reason to suspect that a child or an adult has been harmed or not adequately cared for.

If a physician or healthcare provider does not tell the right people that a child is at risk of being neglected or victimized by abuse, or ignores a child's medical problems, he or she could be arrested, fined, and reported. Medical professionals would then have neglected their healthcare responsibilities to the little child, the parents, the government, and to society. It is everyone's responsibility to protect children. If you know a child who is in serious trouble, you can pick up the telephone and tell someone without having to give your name. The safety and protection of children is a top priority, for all of us.

Keep breathing, my friend, and hang in there. When the disease of alcoholism and drug addiction affects children, healthcare workers pull together information to try to get an idea of the family's situation and the baby's health condition. Healthcare workers notify a child welfare protective agency if they believe a child is in danger of neglect or abuse, or if a family isn't able to adequately care for the baby because of past or present circumstances.

A hospital social worker will complete paperwork that describes the medical conditions and social situations of mother and child. Each important area about the family may be assigned a level of risk for current problems and future events. For example, if mom received prenatal care, she can probably be depended upon to follow through with her child's doctor appointments, and the risk of the baby not getting medical care would be low. If mom is homeless, or if there is drug and alcohol use by someone at home, that is a high risk situation for a baby's future. The hospital social worker usually notes if mom has some support from a relative, such as the father, grandmother, or aunt. If necessary, a telephone call is made and the forms are sent to a child protective services office. The healthcare institution has notified the proper agency, because it's the law.

The hospital does not determine what happens next and cannot make decisions about a child's placement. If your healthcare provider has reasonable suspicion and must report it, this does not mean a child is automatically taken away or removed from mom's custody. The state agency is in charge of checking out the baby's situation. This means a children's welfare worker will be asked to investigate the effects of drug and alcohol dependency on members of a family, including past and present lifestyle, mom's parenting capabilities, baby's condition, and any other factors that may have caused difficulties inside a family, such as domestic violence or sexual abuse.

The child welfare worker's number one job is to make sure babies and other children are safe, cared for, and protected from harm. It may not seem like it, but the worker's number two concern is to keep families together, if at all possible. Professionals realize that children and parents need each other. If a mom with chemical dependency problems receives supportive services, it is often believed to be in the baby's best interests that they remain together for the child's ongoing development.

When the disease of alcoholism and drug addiction impacts mothers and their children, the situation can become confusing and complicated. First of all, knowledge about chemical dependency and infant drug and alcohol exposure is still rather new. More and more information is learned each year about addictive substances, and their effects on adults, children, and whole communities. Second, different individuals have varying beliefs when it comes to issues of addiction. Every state has its own laws and procedures about chemically dependent pregnant women and prenatally exposed infants. By 1994, some states made laws that provided treatment or coordinated services for women; none had passed specific criminal penalties for women whose babies had been prenatally exposed to controlled substances. Third, every mother, child, and family is unique and should be evaluated in terms of their strengths, as well as their weaknesses, for a baby's safety and continuing growth.

Last but not least, professionals want drug- and alcohol-dependent women to be encouraged to get medical care and drug and alcohol treatment for themselves and for their children, rather than being afraid and discouraged from obtaining these lifesaving services. One president of the United States, Bill Clinton, called for more substance abuse treatment programs and better social services to reach out and support pregnant and parenting women. Please know that many people want to help you and your children toward healing the disease of addiction in your family. But the most important person who can improve this situation is you.

A child welfare worker tries to figure out what difficulties can be solved quickly, what counseling services or other referrals a family might need, and which problems will take longer to be corrected. They need to know which factors in a family would not threaten a child's safety, as well as those that could cause abuse or neglect. The main authorities who decide where, when, or for how long a baby may be placed in the custody of someone other than the parent are the state's child welfare agency and juvenile and family civil court.

People who are experienced in perinatal addiction realize that some mothers are capable of properly caring for their exposed babies. But some drug and alcohol addicted mothers do not have the ability to shield their children from neglect or abuse. Child protective agency personnel gather information, interview mothers and others, and evaluate the family's needs, to make a good decision with the baby's best interests in mind. Several examples that help a worker decide on a child's placement is a baby's medical condition; finding out if the mother has already enrolled or is willing to attend a drug and alcohol treatment program, and stick with it; or if a child has a clean, sober, and healthy grandparent who can help.

Children's welfare professionals decide if a family's case should be accepted at all, or if helping the family would be enough to make sure an infant is safe to grow healthier at home. Several options are available for the worker to choose from which should always be the least disruptive for members of a family, and give adequate protection for the baby. Besides, shelter and foster care are expensive and possibly not the greatest places for a child. Drug and alcohol treatment and supportive social services are less costly, and can help families so much, that the hundreds of problems caused by addiction would not have to happen, ever again. Families, like yours and mine, do recover.

If a baby's mother is well and the home is considered safe, the child might remain with her. Mom may be asked by the child's welfare worker to sign a family maintenance agreement that outlines what the agency will do to help, and what mom needs to do to improve herself and the caretaking of her infant and other children. The child welfare worker will assist the family in correcting the problems and preventing new ones that could add up to an abusive or neglectful situation. The worker might refer the family to social services like chemical dependency treatment, domestic violence counseling, or a parenting class. The worker also monitors the healthcare of mom and infant, and tracks the family's progress.

If a family's home and lifestyle are not okay for a baby's safety and healthy development, or cannot be improved enough with a child welfare worker's assistance, a dependency petition will be filed at child and family court. A court date will be scheduled quickly, where the judge closely examines all information, medical and social welfare reports, and talks to mother and family.

The court makes sure that every reasonable effort was made toward strengthening the family. The judge may recommend that the baby remain with mom and more services be provided to the family, or that removal from the family situation would be best for the child.

If not left in a parent's care, the baby will then be in relative custody (with a family member), or in foster care. The child protective services worker will make sure the infant is doing well, and will probably set up a schedule for mom to visit and participate in the baby's care. The placement option of relative custody or foster care is about reunifying the family. The focus is on helping mom and family remove the conditions that could endanger a child. The baby could then be returned sooner, rather than later, to a safe home and a healthy parent.

As time goes on, the child protective agency might decide that a child's family cannot provide the minimum protection for safety, or appropriate food, shelter, parenting, and other requirements. They ask if mom has participated in a good alcohol and drug treatment program and is currently clean and sober, attended parenting classes, or followed through with other recommendations made to her by child welfare. The agency must show that they have made every effort to help the family and resolve the problems that stood in the way of the family being together. The welfare worker's report includes how they worked together with parents, children, and organizations toward reunification. If a child will be in serious danger by being reunified or remaining with a parent, the juvenile dependency judge may seek permanent custody for a child's placement.

Some babies have fallen through the cracks of the system. You deserve to know the truth regarding why state agencies are serious about the care of exposed babies and the lifestyles of their moms. Even though addicted parents do not want their children to be hurt, some mothers and fathers do not realize until it is too late that their addictions can take away their children, forever. A two-week-old baby died from a heart attack caused by mom's cocaine use during pregnancy. An eight-and-a-half-months pregnant woman driving drunk had an accident and miscarried. A child was born brain damaged from drug exposure. A baby's death was caused by his teenage brother's drugs getting into a bottle of milk.

When parents didn't stop using cocaine, a seven-week-old child passed away due to malnutrition and dehydration.

These tragedies happen everywhere, every year. My heart goes out to the moms who allowed the disease of addiction to keep them sick and take over their lives and the lives of their babies. They lingered too long before seeking recovery from drugs and alcohol, and now must climb out of the valley of the shadow of death.

*Don't let this happen to you.*

If you are involved with child protective services, there is much you can do that will benefit your case. Start by healing your own difficulties that keep your family apart. Become honest about what's happening in your life, and open up your heart and your mind. For instance, get into recovery for your alcohol and drug addictions. Try to find a treatment program that specializes in pregnant and parenting women and their families. These perinatal programs will better understand when you need to be absent from treatment, if your baby has a doctor's appointment, or you have a court date. You need only to be responsible, and let your counselor know when and why you are unable to attend that day. Back it up with paper, showing you had an appointment, and give it to your counselor and children's social worker. It'll work for you because you're doing the work.

Keep up with medical checkups for yourself and your children. If you had a cesarean section delivery, the nurse will want to make sure your abdomen (stomach) is healing okay and will probably want to see you within two weeks of delivery. If you delivered vaginally, your postpartum checkup will usually be scheduled about six weeks after the baby's birth. These are important, so don't miss out.

Begin thinking of the best birth control method that would work for you, and talk to the nurse or doctor about it at your postpartum exam. Protection from an unplanned pregnancy and harmful sexually transmitted diseases is a beautiful way to start loving yourself. It would be really hard for any woman to show up consistently for drug and alcohol treatment and other services if she became pregnant again and was at risk for deadly infections.

Women need time and energy to get well. Start by taking care of your body as a way of getting your life together.

Grab some paper and a folder for yourself to keep track of your efforts toward recovery and fulfilling your obligations. You don't have to feel you're doing it for anyone else. You could be doing it for your baby, for you, and for your family's future happiness and togetherness. If your case went to child and family court, keep your minute orders and other paperwork together, and note future court dates and the worker's and investigator's telephone numbers and addresses.

In this time of sadness and confusion, it will be helpful to write down everything you're doing toward helping your baby to be safe and your family to be healthy. Your case with a child welfare agency will be evaluated at regular intervals, like every month or every six months. A lot can happen in six months, so write it down. Putting things on paper is a good idea for anyone, but will be a great help to people who are detoxing from their drug and alcohol use and are newly clean and sober. Don't miss appointments, whether they are for court, healthcare, treatment, or social services. Showing up for your treatment obligations, and having documentation on paper that shows you've been following through, will go a long way toward resolving your case.

If you aren't into recovery activities already, this is the time to show you are ready, willing, and able, to do whatever you need to do to remain together, or to get together, with your baby. If you are getting help to be clean and sober from your addictions, you will form a lasting connection whenever you and your baby are together. You can trust that your love will shine through your problems. Hang in there, and don't disappear if it feels like these problems are drowning you. Keep swimming because I'm rooting and cheering for you, and so is your baby.

Here's another good reason why addicted women need hope for recovery from drug and alcohol abuse. A minority of states have brought unusual charges against women when problems and fetal drug and alcohol exposure have occurred. Criminal courts do direct pregnant and parenting women to chemical dependency treatment through diversion, alternative sentencing, or deferred prosecution, and frown upon incarceration. I care enough to talk to you about the reality of justice court involvement that might, however remotely, happen.

If parents do not find recovery for their addictions after the birth of their child, some infants could be in for sickness and trouble. Legal representatives do not want any baby's situation to end up in tragedy, followed by a court case of abuse or neglect. Superior Court judges want to make good decisions, and actively seek the best direction to take that can help solve problems of substance-exposed children fairly, without creating new ones.

I cannot see how increasing the pain, anger, and shame of chemical dependency with justice proceedings that single out women could have anything but a painful, unhealthy effect on their growing children. Many informed organizations, such as the American Civil Liberties Union, the American Society of Addiction Medicine (see Appendix), and the American Medical Association, have gone on public record saying that they are against the prosecution of pregnant or parenting chemically dependent women because their babies have been prenatally exposed. It has not been proven that an infant's health will improve from criminally penalizing its mother, yet child and family civil court recommendations may benefit children, and their families.

Babies are helped most by helping their mothers, rather than punishing women who are caught in the illness and disease of addiction. Women need to feel safe to talk honestly about drug and alcohol addiction and to seek needed medical and social services, whether they are speaking to doctors, social welfare workers, or court representatives.

Luckily, women have recovered their lives, their health, and their children, no matter what level of involvement they have had with "the system." Every woman deserves opportunities to get well. Judges and social welfare people continue to ask for more programs and better services for women and children. Too few programs work with pregnant women, or have services for kids that enable a mother to complete an effective, time-consuming, top quality drug and alcohol treatment program. But, some terrific programs are out there, and you can use this guide to locate one that would be able to give you what you need—sobriety, serenity, and peace of mind.

Women rarely use legal or illegal drugs and alcohol alone. Nor do they become pregnant on their own. Family-centered substance abuse treatment programs need to be more readily available and include parenting classes and sex education for men and women. If a child's best interest is a state's priority, communities need accessible, effective, affordable childcare for all families, and particularly for those who participate in recovery efforts. Mothers, fathers, and children, who have been harmed by drug and alcohol use, can make many positive contributions to their neighborhoods after a family recovers.

You are needed and wanted, not only by your children, but by your community, to become a woman who brightens the world around her, rather than someone who adds to the dark side of her neighborhood. If you are a woman caught in a web spun by your drug and alcohol abuse, you can feel better and improve your life in a reasonably short time. However long it takes, recovery is worth doing.

Following the delivery of a drug- and alcohol-exposed infant, an addicted woman in California enrolled in a perinatal treatment program. She gained nine months of sobriety from drugs and alcohol, was happy and grateful and sober for the first time at a birthday party for her five-year-old daughter. She is completing her high school education to go on to a vocational rehabilitation class for typing and computers. Her infant daughter and toddler son are also doing great, since mom obtained social services, good medical care, specialized childcare, parenting skills, and recovery tools in the treatment program. Her child welfare case is expected to be closed soon. She helps other addicted women by talking about her recovery experience, going to AA and NA meetings, and remaining clean and sober, and stays close and attentive to her children. She isn't bored, either. She feels really good about herself.

Begin your own story of recovery. Living in fear isn't really living; it's just existing until the next hit, drink, or frightening event. Whether you plan it or fake it, accept that your life is changing, and get help to change it for the better. You can't change the past, but you can clear up the clouds of addiction hanging over your head. You can design a new, surprise ending to the story of your life. I have written that no one has a crystal ball. Well, I do. What I see is ... whatever has happened because of your drug addiction and alcoholism can be used as a springboard for you to dive into a cool, clean, clear, sober life. Your children naturally know how to swim in those waters, and so can you!

# CHAPTER 7

## Special Parenting for Extra-Special Babies

To a baby, you are magic. You make a bottle or a breast appear out of thin air for good food and loving contact. You can change your baby's mood by changing his or her body position, diapering, or singing softly. Giving your extra-special infant the best possible care doesn't require magic, nor is there anything mysterious about learning to properly parent a high risk infant. All it takes is an open mind, a big heart, and a pair of willing hands. There are many tried and true things you can do that will greatly improve your child's natural abilities to grow healthier, happier, and stronger. If you notice your mind slamming shut at these suggestions, pry it open and give them a try.

Many times I have heard excuses from recovering alcoholic and drug-addicted women when they resist or blow off learning a parenting technique that clearly helps their babies. "I only used drugs the first three months." "My baby is just little; he's okay." "I didn't drink through my whole pregnancy." "My other kids are fine." Women who explain their hesitation like this about using specific parenting skills are trying to forget, ignore, or deny that their child has been affected by their addictions.

The truth is your baby needs your help. Period. So leave prejudice behind, see that an easy, simple act of parenting can relieve a lot of distress, congratulate yourself for doing what's best for your baby, and go for it. All you have to gain is a calm, secure, happily growing baby, and good feelings about yourself. Ready? We'll go over some wonderful ways to assist and comfort a baby who has been exposed to drugs and alcohol during prenatal development.

This is a chapter for you to look at again and again. Why? Medical research people who have studied high risk babies have found two things that do more to protect a child from future health and social difficulties than anything else. Having a stable home environment, and being with caregivers who are responsive to a baby's needs can decrease or even resolve some children's physical, mental, and emotional problems caused by drug and alcohol exposure.

A stable environment doesn't change every time a parent struggles or the wind blows. It is consistently nurturing to an infant. You can give this to your baby by making sure you and your home situation are secure, drug-free, alcohol-free, and attentive to a child's needs. By helping your newborn with the suggestions that follow, you can promise your child, and assure yourself, that the months and years ahead will be healthier, more fun, and less stressful.

## The First Six Months

These techniques may seem simple or unusual, but they are effective for infants as they grow to six months of age. Alcohol- and drug-affected newborns do better when their mothers and caretakers use the techniques described below. Focusing on giving your baby exactly what's needed for his or her healthy development will nurture you, too. Being able to answer your baby's distress signals, and watching him or her become cool, calm, and collected will fill you with satisfaction and joy. I know you can do it.

Always show up for your baby's medical appointments. If you are observing and caring for your newborn, you are the best person to tell the doctors and nurses what's happening with your baby. If someone else is taking care of the baby, go along and stay involved. Infant specialists will listen to a caregiver's "baby reports," and together, you and the doctor will discover the best ways to meet your child's needs.

All babies need to be seen by a healthcare provider often for shots that immunize and protect them from serious diseases like polio, measles, diphtheria, and meningitis. These diseases can cause kids to become physically disabled or threaten their survival due to blood, brain, bone, or tissue infections. There are no ifs, ands, or buts about it when it comes to preventing death and disease by getting your child immunized. Children must receive their immunization shots, and must get them according to a specific schedule as they grow.

Newborns will receive some immunizations at the hospital within the first two days of life. Make appointments for your baby at one, two, four, and six months of age for other immunizations. Children need to get these protective medicines on time, until they are sixteen years old. For this reason, have a regular doctor or the same clinic treat your child. Request a little immunization booklet from your doctor so you can keep a record of these medications that save children's lives.

Infants change a lot in six months and the methods that will help them the most can change as your baby grows. Get information and feedback from medical personnel during your baby's checkups. Ask what you can do at any given time in a child's new life that will improve his or her development, and your life together.

The main goal for mothers and others who take care of special babies is to *give them the right kind of attention and stimulation, but not to overstimulate or stress them out, and to know what to do if they become stressed.* Guess who will let you know when he or she is feeling uncomfortable or distressed? Your amazing baby will.

Your job is to learn the clues that will tell you how your infant is managing, moment to moment, and to use these parenting tools to respond to your baby's physical and emotional needs. This is a terrific thing to do because you and your baby will then have longer periods of relating to each other, filled with comfort, security, and contentment. By giving babies your full attention while you care for them, you are letting them know that they are important to you, helping them to feel safe and trusting. What a lovely thing to do for your child.

Your infant could need many of these techniques or just a few to insure its continuing health, and may need them for a few weeks or for many months. Every baby is a little individual person who will enjoy some things more than others, and will prefer a certain way of being held, talked to, or fed, to remain secure in its new environment outside of the womb. Try them all; find out which ones work best for your little person.

Your baby will develop more survival skills and learn at a faster rate now than at any other time. Meeting our goal of helping sensitive babies grow and learn about the world without letting the environment overwhelm them can be pretty tricky. Infants need a variety of sounds, sights, and activities to stimulate the mental and physical processes of learning. Listening to mom talk, sing, hum, and laugh, or looking at colorful pictures and interesting shapes gives babies enjoyment as well as the important learning and language experiences they need. However, when their calm, alert interest turns into nervousness and distress, start thinking about these parenting skills.

A baby must have a mother or primary caregiver who is emotionally available, answering calls for food, comfort, or companionship. Which type of person would you rather be with? Someone who approaches you with a gentle smile, a soft voice, and soothing touches, or someone who comes at you with loud, barking sounds, an upset face, and sharp, impatient movements? Which kind of person would help you eat, sleep, and communicate better? If you were crying and hungry, wet, or anxious, would you trust someone who came every time, or who only came to help you part of the time? I thought you'd say that, and your baby would say the same thing.

At first, your baby may only be able to stay calm and attentive while being talked to or handled for short periods of time. The world is often a confusing place and even a caregiver's face can seem overwhelming to look at, listen to, and interact with. *At all times, watch your baby for these behaviors that signal an infant is over-stimulated and stressed:*

- avoiding eye contact—moves head to the side, or looks away during interactions with people or things in their field of vision

- tension—easily startled, arching the spine, throwing the head back, frantic crying or sucking, shakiness

- frowning and grimacing—scrunching up the face, maybe closing the eyes, face becoming anxious (watch the eyebrows)

- yawning and sneezing—open mouth, moving head, seeming to gasp

- sucking on hands and fingers—let them do it; this comforts infants and they learn about their bodies and safe movements

The more you see, recognizing the clues and responding to a baby's subtle, quiet signals of stress, as well as obvious, distressed crying, the healthier your child will be. Children will then develop a trusting bond with you. For example, an exposed infant can feel frightened and confused from sounds, faces, and being touched when it's all happening at the same time. Quieting the home environment and the people in it, holding your child properly to decrease a stimulating event, and giving a baby time to regroup emotionally will enable the baby to stay attentive to you and learn at his or her own pace. This is a very loving, respectful way to treat your baby.

Learning to correctly handle, hold, and position vulnerable babies is certain to help them grow emotionally and physically. Just like you, infants experience many feelings throughout the day, such as irritability, pleasure, and fear. They need you to support their body posture, muscle tone, and emotional states while sleeping, carrying, and feeding, in order to stay calm. Relaxed babies eat more, sleep better, and have less stomach and bowel problems. They can then gain weight consistently, and be ready to play more often, responding easily to your smile and touch.

Remember that chemicals affect an infant's central nervous system, the brain and the spinal cord. Your child may have tense muscles, an arched back, overextended neck, and legs and arms that have been outstretched for long periods of time. Or, a baby could have little muscle tone, and be moving its head and limbs in a floppy manner. You can increase healthy growth and comfort by using a receiving blanket to keep your baby's body curved in a more natural position, with bent arms and legs kept closer to the midsection. Exposed babies may not be able to do this on their own, and need your reassurance and a snug blanket wrapped securely around them to help their bodies relax.

Swaddling gives infants control over their movements, allowing them to better organize their bodies and their emotions, and decreases jitteriness and irritability. So let's do it. Lay your baby facing you on a soft receiving blanket with the head in one corner. If it's a hot time of year, you can use a small, light crib sheet. Bend an arm at the elbow, leg at the knee, and wrap that side of the blanket around the baby securely, putting the limbs (arms and legs) next to his or her body. Bring up the bottom corner of the blanket, making sure the legs are bent at the knees. Then wrap the other side, as if you were folding a tortilla around to make a burrito. The baby's hands must be free, close enough to reach the mouth, while the elbows are held by the blanket next to the baby's body. Make sure baby's hip area is comfortably bent.

Think of helping your baby grow by curving his or her body like it was inside the womb. Wrap the swaddling blanket snug but not too tight so the chest can expand, making breathing easy. Keep an infant's nostrils clear of mucus, breast milk, or dried formula since a stuffy nose also restricts a baby's breathing.

If an infant is shaky or hard to soothe when laid down to sleep, swaddle in a blanket and put the baby on his or her side. Place a rolled up cloth diaper or towel next to the back, along the spine. The support roll of cloth behind the back will help the baby stay in this side-lying position. Babies should have enough freedom to move their legs, and hands in front of them to reach their mouth. If your child doesn't appear to like being swaddled at night, you can put a rolled up cloth diaper along the back, and one between its bent legs. Then place a light blanket up to the shoulders, and tuck it securely under the mattress on both sides. This also helps a baby's body remain in a supported, curved side-lying posture but relaxes tremors, muscle stiffness, and controls floppy movements, which keep infants awake and struggling.

You are learning what to do when your baby is irritable, stressed out, and hard to console or soothe. If, at any time, your calming techniques like swaddling, changing body positions, singing, or pacifying don't work right away, take a deep breath. If you find yourself becoming angry, sweaty, or panicked, lay your swaddled baby comfortably and safely in the crib, and back away for a three-minute break. You are human, and at moments when it feels like it's too much, put the baby down, and recognize that you're both having a rough day. Take just a few minutes and go brush your hair, read a funny comic, or enjoy a recovery book with your feet up. Knowing when you need to cool out is an essential parenting skill.

The greatest mothers have nerves, too, and need to give themselves permission to pause, get a grip on their emotions, call someone, or find a sitter and go for a half-hour walk. Three to five minutes alone can make a big difference in helping tired, shattered moms regain their patience and spirit. Don't take your human, adult-sized frustration out on a scattered infant. Take a short break and relax instead, okay? This would be a caring thing to do for yourself and your baby.

Your infant might relax into sleep faster if you drape a light cloth on the side of the crib (but not over it). This way, a baby won't become distracted and anxious from seeing people or a confusing room full of strange shadowy shapes. When it's time for babies to rest, keeping their sleeping area quiet, less bright, warm, and visually soothing is best. Don't forget the pacifier.

Knowing the normal sleep pattern for an infant is really important. You will know if you should worry and if you need to tell your pediatrician that your baby is having trouble falling asleep, staying asleep, or sleeping too much. First, babies and adults awaken frequently, up to four times a night. We don't remember waking up because older people have learned to soothe themselves and relax back to sleep. Babies are just learning to do this. Second, it takes an average of twenty-seven minutes for an infant to fall asleep. You don't have to panic if your baby needs almost a full half-hour to go to sleep. It's normal for newborns to sleep a short time, and be awake for short periods of time. Third, as children get older, they need less time to calm themselves into restful sleep.

By using your new parenting techniques from this chapter, you can help your baby sleep more comfortably and develop a more normal sleeping schedule. You will also feel less frustrated when a little one awakens after several hours and needs your care. When babies grow to three months of age, they will be awake longer and sleep more, up to about four hours. Most six-month-old babies sleep about six hours at a time. Now you'll sleep better, too.

Only swaddle-wrap infants when they need it to calm down in order to eat, sleep, or stay relaxed yet alert when awake. Babies will gradually gain an ability to relax themselves since you've been doing a great job helping them by swaddling, positioning, and watching for overstimulation clues from their face and body motions. When infants can calmly and actively respond without needing assistance, they will then be ready to go on to new learning adventures.

Restrict uncontrollable movements when necessary, but also provide opportunities for growth and discovery, like letting infants push themselves up while lying on their stomachs. An unbreakable mirror, securely fastened at eye level, will encourage your child to raise up on elbows and see the cute baby looking back. Or, draw a smiley face on paper and tape it to the crib. If your baby sends distress signals from looking at his or her reflection or a picture, respond by comforting baby, taking it down, and trying again in a few weeks. Let babies be your guide when it comes to new experiences: remember almost everything is new to them!

When feeding, carrying, and holding vulnerable infants, keep them close, held firmly against your body. You will be helping small babies to develop trust in you and in the people who care for them. During moments of stress from too much activity, quickly place the infant against your shoulder facing behind you, or put baby's back securely against your chest, facing forward. Infants also do well if you carry them in the crook of your arm with baby's arms in front to reach and grab, and bent legs supported by your arm and hands. For all of these positions, support baby's body, keeping knees and hips bent, arms in front, and eyes gazing away from faces and places that can cause too much excitement and stress. There's always the front pack carrier to strap on if you need a free hand, and baby can rest against your chest.

If your little one begins to show signs of tension, such as not looking into your eyes or an arched back, start to decrease the effects of overstimulation by changing your baby's body position and swaddling. Letting nervous infants relax by staring into the distance really helps them since newborns can focus on confusing faces and objects that are about a foot away from them. After babies have collected their anxious emotions and you feel their bodies relax, you can slowly place them face to face for a quiet conversation. Help them to trust and get to know your voice and touch by holding them firmly, stroking their face gently, and speaking tenderly.

Slow, easy rocking and soft, consistent sounds from you can quickly stop a baby's crying and relax a child, so the two of you can visit. Your baby would probably enjoy gentle up and down rocking while being held in a vertical (head up) position. Avoid side to side motions because fast, horizontal movements can cause a baby to become disoriented and fearful. As a child's loving protector, don't let anyone, even brothers and sisters, bounce, swing, sharply pat, or roughly handle your sensitive baby.

Forget baby walkers, and only use swings and jumpers with extreme caution. If you have a walker, give it away or put it away. Walkers can actually delay a child's walking skills, because while using them infants tend to stay stiff in their legs, back, hip area, and neck. To push themselves forward, babies learn to walk on their toes rather than balancing on both feet. High risk infants need to get a good crawl going first, moving their bodies in a flexed, organized fashion, before learning to walk.

When using swings or jumpers, mom needs to remain close to avoid accidents; never leave baby alone in equipment that moves. A baby's head and neck need to be supported while in a swing or jumper, and swinging motions can confuse an infant's delicate nervous system. Watch your baby for signs of overstimulation to see if she or he is soothed from the repetitive movement, or is fighting the motion and feeling stress and discomfort.

Many substance-exposed infants like to stand at an early age and be able to stretch their muscles. Just like helping babies to be flexible for healthier bone, muscle, and nerve growth, you can support them while they stand with feet flat on the floor or on your lap, but only for very small amounts of time. *The muscles are not strong, but tense,* and their bodies need plenty of relaxation to avoid muscle strain and fatigue (overtiredness).

If your infant is stressed and it's not time to sleep, soft, rhythmic music may be soothing to your baby. During a bath, diaper change, or while cradled in your lap, gentle, steady massage that relaxes nerves and muscles might help your baby return to a calm, alert state. Remove your jewelry and make sure the room is warm. Start by talking to your baby, asking if touching feels okay, and gently massage the chest and stomach in slow circles. Massage the arms, legs, back, and buttocks in long, easy strokes. Watch your infant to discover the firmness of your touch that he or she likes best and continue. Or notice the signs of distress, then stop and swaddle-wrap.

If your baby responds well, start by massaging for a few minutes every other day, then gradually increase the length of time. When premature or full-term infants are carefully and regularly massaged, they improve in weight gain, blood circulation, skin condition, and the functioning of their nervous systems from mom's healing touch. Organs and muscles are nourished from massage, becoming flexible and vigorous. Use oil or baby lotion, warm up your hands, and caress your baby to health.

The television is lousy company for a baby. The constant sound and quickly changing pictures become too much, making infants work hard to shut them out. Besides, televisions cannot respond to your baby the way you can, so if you're watching the tube, place your baby in front, facing you.

Keep a pacifier on hand and let your infant relax by sucking, giving baby time to collect scattered emotions. Most babies need to satisfy their sucking reflex even when they are not hungry because it releases tension. Mothers with inquiring minds need to know when baby wants to eat, or just needs to suck and relax.

Feeding can sometimes be troublesome for drug- and alcohol-affected infants. Take all the time necessary for your baby to comfortably breathe, suck, and swallow, so the liquid can flow easily down the throat, into the stomach, and not come back up. If your baby is sucking anxiously and frantically, help him or her to relax by swaddling, comforting, waiting, and burping often, to avoid spitting up. To keep air from being swallowed, which causes stomach pain, hold your baby in a semi-upright position during feeding.

Try not to become impatient at baby's mealtime. Your child may only be able to swallow a little formula or breast milk (like an ounce) at a time and will need to be fed more often and at regular intervals. Feed babies on schedule, and don't let them go for more than four hours without eating. Many babies are sensitive to formulas, and may or may not need extra iron. If you're not breast-feeding, always check with the doctor or nurse to find the formula that nourishes your infant the best.

The only liquids babies should have are breast milk or formula, and perhaps plain water. If your child is four months or younger, give 'em kisses, but don't give your little one soda, sweetened drinks, cereal, or anything else he or she shouldn't have in a bottle. A vulnerable baby should not have a bottle propped up with the nipple stuck in his or her mouth and be left all alone. Your baby needs to gaze into your eyes, hear your soft, friendly voice, feel your comforting arms, and not choke or gag on formula or breast milk. Why? Because baby is learning now, as well as eating, enjoying, and growing.

Babies learn to trust their mothers and caregivers when adults respond immediately to their needs for food, comfort, and love. No matter what anybody says or who says it, it is impossible to spoil a baby under one year old. *Impossible.* If you comfort crying, anxious newborns for several months, these babies will cry less later on and be able to soothe themselves more often, because you helped them feel secure when they were younger. Don't let your baby continue to cry, remain in a soiled diaper, or feel hunger, loneliness, or stress. Infants cannot make it alone, and your special child depends on your tender loving care to grow normally or to catch up in development. Now is the time to show your child that the world is an okay place, and that you are a caring, attentive person who is trustworthy and safe to be with.

Newborns will turn their heads in the direction of their mother's voice while in the womb and after birth. When mom talks, baby listens. Here's your chance to be a star with a captive audience, so sing, hum, talk, and share stories to your heart's content. Why? You can help develop a child's social skills, self-confidence, and even increase the level of intelligence. How? By talking, singing, explaining, and reading to your little baby.

We don't usually have to pay people to talk to a baby. Adults enjoy repeating baby's sounds and naturally mimic an infant's goos and gaas, sighs and grunts. And the baby is delighted. Hanging out with adults and learning to be social becomes more fun. The little one has found that she or he can communicate with these big people and have some impact on the conversation. When mom repeats baby's sounds, babies talk more because they are rewarded with her attention, affection, and more sounds. You will be blessed with the gifts of your baby's love, interest, and healthy development of language, by talking to your little child.

If your infant is not regularly vocalizing by crying, babbling, or turning toward your voice, make a doctor's appointment because these could be warning signs of an early speech or hearing problem. Tell your infant medical specialist what you've observed, and don't panic. When it comes to language development, quick detection and good care can prevent a speech disorder later.

Infants learn to talk and feel free to express themselves because they are spoken to with love and respect. If you're a woman who is shy and often inside of herself, make a special effort to talk and verbalize lots of sounds to your baby. Bring the baby into your world by talking about the home you share or how you feel while fixing dinner or changing a diaper. If you are naturally an outgoing, talkative person, you may need to watch your infant more closely to know when to pause, talk less, or speak more softly.

Continue to watch for signs of stress from your baby during your conversations. If his or her eyes look away from you, if baby is sucking on his or her fingers or frowning, take a break from the discussion and let your baby rest by changing his or her position (held against your shoulder, in the crook of your arm, or against your chest, facing outward). From reading this chapter on parenting skills carefully, and using these tools for your baby's healthy development, you will know what to do for your baby, when to do it, and you will enjoy doing it more! Wow—you are something! Keep reading.

Whether speaking, singing, or play-talking, mom becomes baby's first language teacher. Hearing her voice comforts a baby, and listening to the different words teaches little ones about their world. For example, babies need to hear you say "hello" and "good-bye" and talk or sing songs about bedtime or bathtime. From hearing these special sounds, infants begin to understand that mom is coming, going, and will come back again. They'll recognize from your voice that it's time to sleep, eat, or bathe. Use lots of little words and songs with your baby because you are helping to prepare your baby for what's going to happen next. So, hearing the sounds and learning that certain words mean something is about to happen creates security and happiness in a child's heart. Even though they are little babies, believe it—they understand.

Not many of us like painful surprises, especially when mom disappears and reappears without warning, or infants suddenly find themselves in a tub of water. Being steady and consistent in telling your baby what you're doing, and what they'll be doing, gives children time to prepare themselves emotionally. Infants will be less frightened of the changes taking place. You will hear a lot less crying when you leave the room or get ready to go out, say, to a treatment group, recovery meeting, or your postpartum checkup.

What do you think is the best, most important thing you can do for your baby's mental development and later, greater success in life? Now I'm going to surprise you. The answer is reading out loud. When do you think would be the best time to start reading to your child? Age two, three, or four? Now we're both surprised. Start reading aloud to your infant now, or at least by four months of age. Along with bonding in the warmth of your arms and the security of your voice, babies are learning language, coordinating movements, and developing eyesight by seeing colors and shapes as the pages are turned.

Reading aloud is the perfect opportunity to teach your baby so many things. When you point to a picture of a cat, you can say what it is, if the kitty has a name, make a cat sound, explain the tail and eyes and point out the ears and whiskers. Would this cat scratch or bite? Pretty important information for children to know. And you will be giving it to them.

Your baby is constantly learning. Anytime your baby is in one place, like in the crib, on the floor, or in a playpen, put up a bright mobile if your baby enjoys it without feeling stressed. Music boxes, small bells, or homemade rattles are interesting sounds to infant ears. Put magazine pictures in baby's places at eye level, and re-place them often. Interesting things to hold, like a furry stuffed animal and a soft quilt, help a child's sense of touch. Give infants safe items to grab for, like rattles and plastic dishes. Nothing too small should be within a baby's reach or go into a child's mouth. If you are unsure of feeding times or safe toys, concerned about de-pressed emotions, jitteriness, overexcited crying, diaper rash, or anything else that affects your little one, talk to the right people, ask questions, and ask them often.

You are a rainbow of hope in your child's life if you are recov-ering from drug and alcohol addiction. You will also be worth more than a pot of gold if you are using these suggestions for parenting and caring for your infant. Babies are individuals with their own strengths, as well as weaknesses. See their strengths, watch for weaknesses, and start from there. Insisting your child be different from who he or she really is enables moms to shrug off and avoid caring for their baby's specific problems. Mothers who are not attentive to their children's development will also lose out on the joy of celebrating their children's successes.

## Respect and Expectations

It's very important to have the right idea about what children can and cannot do. Many women, some of whom have older children, are often unrealistic in what they expect their baby to do, what their baby should do for them, or what they expect from them-selves. Unrealistic expectations mean wanting something to hap-pen or not happen which isn't possible and couldn't become real.

What would happen if a mother expected her newborn to sleep for eight hours every night, or never cry? This would be unrealistic, because we now know the normal sleep and emotional patterns of infants. It would be impossible, unreasonable, and even cruel to demand that a baby sleep eight hours straight, or not cry. If mom expected this, she might become angry at her baby for sleeping only three hours or crying a few minutes, thinking the infant was being bad or disobedient, call the baby rotten names, or punish the baby. And the baby was just being a real baby.

*Don't let this happen to you! Your baby is worth loving, just as you are.*

Learning about motherhood means respecting children's limitations, as well as your own. Sometimes infants cannot do what you want or expect, not because they are bad, but because they're young, maybe sick, and always need some help. Expecting too much from either of you would be painful to the baby and stressful for you. Parents who do not have a good understanding about what is normal and possible for a child to do, or what would be impossible behavior for a child, too often end up emotionally hurting or physically abusing their children. Babies and moms deserve to be loved for who they are, supported to overcome problems, and congratulated for their healthy development.

Having realistic expectations of yourself as you care for a drug- and alcohol-exposed infant is good for you, too. Mothers who expect the impossible from themselves will find that they don't measure up, because no one is perfect. They begin to dislike caring for their kids, feel inadequate, and move away emotionally from their children when they should be getting closer. Parents do not need to be perfect to improve a child's health, just good enough, by knowing what to do and doing it when babies need assistance.

What's realistic is believing that accidents can happen, and understanding what you can do to prevent your baby from having one. While growing to six months of age, babies are at a high risk for choking, hitting their heads, burns, and poisoning. In no time at all, infants learn to push with their feet, wave their arms, wiggle around, or suddenly roll over. Don't leave your baby, even for one minute, on a high place such as a changing table, bed, or high chair. Pick up small objects left on the floor, and make sure dangerous poisons are already put away in a high cupboard. Use an infant car seat with your baby strapped in tight every time you travel. It's the law in most states, and car crashes are one of the biggest dangers to children's lives.

Many infants suffer burns from waving their fists and knocking over a hot cup of coffee, or grabbing panhandles from the stove. Keep all boiling liquids far away from baby's reach. Don't forget to check the batteries in household smoke alarms. Your child will be safer because you are aware of how life-threatening accidents happen and will protect your infant from everyday injuries.

If you follow these special parenting guidelines for extra-special babies, you will have no reason to feel inadequate or not good enough. The best way to stay close and attentive to your baby's needs is to be there in body, mind, and spirit, and to stay realistic in what you expect from yourself, and from the littlest member of your family. Motherhood—you can give an outstanding, stellar performance, and watch your baby become a star!

# CHAPTER 8

# Recovery:
# A Plan for Living and Loving

*Hi. My name is Yvonne, and I'm an alcoholic and an addict. I have a sixteen-month-old son, and I'm pregnant now. It's a girl. Today is the best day of my life, because I've been clean and sober for exactly one year! Even though I'm scared and running around like a chicken with my head cut off most of the time, I have hope, and my life is better than it's ever been. I don't want to die anymore. I can face my day and my son and my pregnancy without getting fucked up behind drugs and alcohol and my son's father, because I get a lot of help and support. I couldn't do it on my own. Thank God I didn't have to 'cause I never would have made it. But I'm making it now! Just one day at a time, and now I've got a year.*

*My son was still shaky and crying all the time since he was born. I saw a doctor a couple of times when I was pregnant with him, but never went back for lab tests because I was afraid. I was strung out on cocaine, smoking it while my boyfriend was always yelling at me, telling me he was going* to call the police. He had a pipe in one hand, and a beer in the other. And I was supposed to go to a treatment program. When I went to the emergency room, my membranes had ruptured, I was freaking, and they did an emergency C-section to save my son. He was blue when he came out, and pretty small. I was so scared. My boyfriend wasn't even there.

My baby went to my mother's and even though I was glad he wasn't in foster care, he was being treated the same way I was. She didn't pay much attention and cursed at him, and he's only a baby! My mom's still pretty bitter about life, and was really pissed off when child protective services called her. She hadn't heard from me in months.

The court said go to a program, and a parenting class, and get help. I'd visit my baby; he'd be like flying through the air, arms and legs all over the place, jittery, burping up his milk, and my mom would tell me if I didn't get a job she wouldn't want me coming over. How could I get a job when all I could do was hustle my drugs, fight with my boyfriend, and get drunk?

The hospital called me, and a nice lady asked me if I was thinking about getting into a drug and alcohol treatment program. She said there was a place that, if I got custody, I could bring my son with me, because he needed me, and probably could use more help, too. She said other women with the same problem I had were getting well, it was cheap, and then she said . . . they could help me become the mom I always wanted to be. Just come check it out.

We lost our apartment. I wouldn't see my boyfriend for days because he wouldn't come home and when he did, it was bad. I had lost my house, my guy, and my baby. Nobody wanted to see me anymore unless I gave them ass, grass, or money.

I showed up at the treatment program for my appointment. The counselor shook my hand, gave me a cup of coffee, didn't even look at me funny 'cause I hadn't had a shower, and we talked. We talked about addiction. She said it wasn't my fault. But it was my responsibility to get well, and they'd help me. I was afraid, because I didn't trust anybody. But my baby was in the hospital because he couldn't keep his milk *down. Something was wrong with his stomach. I signed papers, giving permission for treatment. The counselor got me into a women's shelter for the night and I could show up for treatment the next day. She knew, and I knew, that I wouldn't make it if I didn't have a safe place to sleep.*

*My baby's social worker told me I had to complete a program, get clean tests, and learn parenting stuff. The shelter said they'd keep me if I went to the program Monday through Friday. At treatment, they fed me lunch and snacks, helped me get financial assistance and a postpartum checkup. I got medicine for an infection I didn't even know I had, and some birth control. I met some women at the treatment program, and now I have friends. Good friends. They took me to meetings. AA and NA meetings, and we laughed a lot. I'd visit my baby and wrap him up and feed him properly and my mom was just amazed. He'd stop crying and calm down, cooing and looking at me. I was so happy I could help him. He was hurtin', too.*

*We had groups at the treatment center—sitting in a circle, talking about our lives and our problems and how to change 'em. When other girls said they were an addict and alcoholic, I could too. Then somebody offered me a rock on the street. I said "Hell no," and got back to the shelter. Man, was I surprised. I guess I felt like something, felt better about myself. My counselor said, I don't have to earn my wings to heaven, just start backing away from hell! And, if I didn't get recovery at the AA meetings and going to outpatient treatment, my life would get worse.*

*I just kept showing up; it got better. I started talking about my feelings. Phew. I had a lot of feelings going on, but I just hung in there, talked about 'em, and didn't act on them. I guess drugs and alcohol kicked my butt enough that I was willing to do what they said, to follow directions. Even when my head told me to go get high, I'd call somebody or read or go to a meeting, and the feeling would pass, just like they said it would, and I had another day of sobriety.*

*I graduated from the treatment program and they had a cake for me and my mom came and my son was there. My dad came and I hadn't seen him in years, and he said he was proud of me. We didn't hug then, but we do now. He goes to AA, too. God, my son is doing so great that the doctor said he'd be ready for preschool soon. When he gets hyper, I know how to help him and calm him down and teach him how to talk about what he wants, so he doesn't have to kick me or throw a tantrum. I tell him I love him and I back it up—he believes what he sees, not what I say. Just like his mom! I haven't left him, I've been there for him and we're pretty close.*

*I treat him the way I want to be treated, with patience and respect. Or else he'll end up like his father, who's still loaded and doesn't know right from wrong. I think he's in jail. I want my son to be nice to women and get along with people so that's what I teach him. I never want my son to go to jail. And I know I don't want my daughter to have to do all the things I did when I was drinking and using.*

*I go to AA and NA meetings all the time. My son is doing okay and I got a neat sober babysitter 'til he starts preschool. I used birth control for a year, then I fell in love, and, oh, well, we'll work it out. Because we're both clean and sober and working a recovery program. You better believe I'm getting prenatal care now. I go back every month to the treatment center and talk to the new girls. I'm told that if I forget where I came from, what my life used to be like drinking and using, I'll go back there. So I tell my story and remind myself that I'm an addict and an alcoholic with a short memory. I used to think I was crazy or a loser, so why try? But I'm just a drug addict and an alcoholic, and there's always more to learn. I still make mistakes but it's no big deal, as long as I'm in recovery. Finally, I can be human. My life is better than it's ever been, and I like who I am today. And I'm a damn good mom, too.*

*Love, Yvonne*

Women need hope when they have felt helpless to change their lives, and help to meet their special emotional, social, spiritual, and physical needs. Let the people in the programs show you the simple tools that have worked for other alcoholic and drug-addicted women. If they can do it, I believe you can too. In healing a life torn apart by substance abuse, there's the inside story, and the outside story.

Fear, inadequacy, anger, and guilt are part of the inside story, and individuals familiar with recovery will comfort and support you as good and not-so-good feelings arise. The outside story is learning to cope with the people, places, and things in your life in a different way, far away from drugging and drinking. Chemically dependent people often keep their anger inside, and turn it against themselves. You don't have to get high or hurt yourself again, or your children, because of how you're feeling or what you're thinking. The tools for living clean and sober, slowly but surely, will give you peace, and you'll be able to create a good life for yourself and your kids.

The choice, between getting treatment for drug addiction and alcoholism while you're hot or continuing to use substances until you're cold, is in your hands and within your power. You are the only person with the power to change your life, make a decision, and go for it. It seems impossible that anyone could truly love themselves or their kids if they're still getting loaded. And everyone wants and needs to be loved, especially mothers and children.

Most addicted persons have followed the "sin now, pray later" plan. If your heart is spiritually inclined, feel free to say a quick prayer for choosing recovery over drug addiction and drunkenness. Otherwise, you're left with the "pay now and pay later" drinking and using plan, which will result in the destruction of all good things: you, your family, and your life. You don't deserve to pay the ultimate price for feeling lost, hopeless, or helpless from having been shackled to drugs and alcohol. You can give yourself what you are entitled to—love. And the people in recovery programs will care about you and treat your disease of addiction until you can love and care about yourself.

You can't scare addicts or alcoholics into doing good things for themselves, but we know that addicted people, without recovery, will eventually lose their lives. How? Chemically dependent people will end up institutionalized, incarcerated, or dying before their time if they don't find a way to live without drugs and alcohol. Mothers become lost to their children. Children are left by the side of the road as parents speed down the highway of drug and alcohol dependency, only to find a dead end.

Some researchers wanted to know what happened to mothers after they delivered children with fetal alcohol syndrome, caused by mom drinking beer, wine, or liquor during pregnancy. Within five years after the birth of their children, 75 percent of these moms were discovered to have died, or were missing in action, unable to be found by their families, friends, or society. These were not bad women; they were sick women who couldn't get well.

You are not a bad person to have survived until now by using drugs and drinking alcohol. It doesn't even matter whether a woman believes substances are her main problem or not. If you think getting money, fighting with your partner, struggling with your kids, feeling ill or depressed, or going to school or work are bigger problems in your life than drinking and using, you can accept chemical dependency treatment, and get help for everything. Making a decision that can turn the painful past into years of future happiness is what matters. If you're using drugs and drinking alcohol, and you are pregnant or have children already, recovery from chemicals is the only way to go. It is the solution to the problem of living for every addict and alcoholic.

Millions of women and men have successfully recovered from the disease of addiction by completing a formal treatment program and by attending Alcoholics Anonymous or Narcotics Anonymous twelve-step programs. Either one can work for you, but your successful recovery depends on your willingness to change your life, and having both feet in a program.

People with one foot in the door and one foot in the street usually find themselves walking away from a clean and sober life, since drugs and alcohol have a powerful pull. Addicts and alcoholics need all their energy to be centered in one place, and if it's not focused on a recovery plan, it'll be on the booze and the drugs. Hop off the fence, plant both feet in a program, and sow the seeds for your new life. If you are an addict and an alcoholic, I know you have the guts to overcome obstacles that block your path, so all you need is the support and guidance of others to find the way.

It takes time to put together a new life full of fun, purpose, play, and recovery to replace the old patterns of using drugs and drinking alcohol. You can find the patience to hang in there by seeing the power that addictive substances had over your spirit. The goal of treatment is to stop using chemicals, learn skills to avoid relapse, and change your life's direction from going down-hill to up, up, and away!

Here's the plan: first, get treatment to stabilize your life and stop all alcohol and drug use. Become connected to a counselor, a chemical dependency doctor, and a bunch of clean and sober people. Learn about the diseases of alcoholism and drug addiction. Get a personal support system together, like a treatment program, twelve-step recovery meetings, maybe your family. Get a health-care provider, trustworthy childcare, a drug-free and alcohol-free place to live, and other services you may need.

As fantasy, denial, and guilt fade away, replace them with a new identity: *a recovering woman with beauty and dignity*. Discover for yourself the benefits of being clean and sober, and watch your inner life and outer circumstances improve. Learn how to make positive choices in your life and relax. Accept that sometimes it's not easy, but it's worth it, because you're worth it, even when you don't think you are. Change your addictive beliefs into recovery thinking, and get lots of help and support to do it. Know the people, places, and things that can cause you to relapse back into drugging and drinking. Stay involved in recovery efforts that make you feel good and move toward peace, in your mind and in your soul.

One way to begin would be to enroll yourself in a chemical dependency treatment program. The women and men who make it are those who remain in a program for at least three months, after choosing a live-in residential program or participating in good outpatient treatment for at least nine hours each week. Mothers who were successful in their recovery had a good relationship with their treatment counselor, and had put together a support system of people who helped them balance out the emotional ups and downs of learning to live free from drugs and alcohol. So, a key to unlocking the chains of addiction seems to be staying in treatment for a minimum of three months and hooking up with a treatment professional you can trust and respect, and joining twelve-step recovery groups.

For example, a mom or a mother-to-be may need a seven-day medical detox, then go to a residential program to stabilize hous-ing or her emotions for thirty days, three months, or more. After gaining her health and strength in recovery, she could attend a perinatal outpatient treatment program that had childcare. She could be reunified with her children before, during, or after treatment, depending on her situation, or following the delivery of a beautiful baby. She would enjoy parenting more, have help with her children and recovery issues, and a place to meet other recovering women.

Remembering the dreams she had, her interests in life, a clean and sober woman could later obtain education or employment. Vocational rehabilitation, job training, GED classes, or other schools would help her do the things she's always wanted to do. As a recovering woman and mother, she would have the gentle encouragement and strong, loving support of her treatment counselor and twelve-step friends as she puts her new life and her family together.

You are not alone. Each year, more than one million women in the United States receive chemical dependency treatment in state funded programs. Most women in treatment today are between the ages of twenty-five and thirty-four. You've tried hard to be happy, to change your life; now you can try something different to accomplish your goal. I know you know, but here goes—keep reading. You're on your way.

Many women are asked to attend and complete a drug and alcohol treatment program, particularly if they are involved with child protective services, child and family court, or other civil or criminal courts. State agencies ask people to participate in treatment programs so that an addict and alcoholic's progress in recovery, and his or her drug- and alcohol-free status, can be confirmed by a treatment facility. If you have a case with one or more of these state agencies, you may be given treatment places to check out, or you can definitely find one that feels okay and right for you by using the referral numbers in the back of this guide.

## Choosing the Right Program

Alcohol and drug treatment programs come in several different flavors, and the most important ingredient is that you pick one and hang in there for three months or more. You want to find a program that will be strong enough to help you fight your fatal attraction to chemicals, but gentle enough so you won't feel you're in the wrong place. Choosing the right type of treatment also depends on the substances you use, whether these chemicals are heroin, prescription drugs, alcohol, cocaine, amphetamines, marijuana, or whatever. A recipe for success is to match your individual needs with the right kind of treatment. Get your taste buds ready, and let's go through your options.

Medical detoxification is needed for people who, because of how much, how long, and which substances they have used, are at risk for big problems during withdrawal. Their bodies have become so dependent upon the chemical, that stopping use would endanger their lives. Some alcoholics, opiate (heroin) addicts, pill (tranquilizers, barbiturates) addicts, and others need to be seen by a treatment professional or a doctor to help them decide if a medical detox is necessary to abstain from substances and begin their recovery.

During this type of treatment, healthcare people watch over an addict and an alcoholic as they come down from intoxication, monitoring their heartbeat, blood pressure, and other vital signs, to avoid physical trauma, hallucinations (DT's), or harming themselves during withdrawal. If needed, the doctor will prescribe medication, and other healthcare measures, to ease symptoms with twenty-four hour, round-the-clock care. Alcohol- and drug-dependent individuals will be more comfortable, able to withdraw safely, and will have their recovery made possible because their poor health and addiction to chemicals were managed in a kind, medically appropriate way.

People at risk for medical complications when withdrawing from substances are usually treated in hospitals, chemical dependency units, and outpatient clinics or programs. Medical detox can last twenty-four hours, three days, two weeks, or longer, depending on the person and the detox program.

As you have read, special detox treatment is really important for some pregnant addicts and alcoholics because of possible medical problems for mom and her developing baby during physical withdrawal. If this is your situation, start with a prenatal care checkup right away to stabilize your health condition. Then, work with your doctor, hospital social worker, or treatment professional, to help you enroll in a detox program that will give a pregnant woman the best care.

Heroin and other opiate-addicted women might choose to withdraw from these substances by attending an outpatient (go to everyday) or inpatient (live-in) methadone program. Methadone keeps them from going into painful withdrawal without becoming high or intoxicated. As their illegal (opiate, cocaine, marijuana) and legal (alcohol or pill) drug use stops, the methadone dose can be decreased until they are feeling comfortable and become physically detoxed. Opiate addicts who have had the greatest success staying drug-free are those who completed a recovery program at a detox clinic, treatment center, or therapeutic community, as well as attending self-help groups, while leaving their opiate addiction and methadone treatment behind. Formerly addicted women can then continue their recovery, free from loneliness and isolation, as they merge into family and community life.

## Inpatient Programs

Many pregnant and parenting women choose a residential drug and alcohol treatment program. They move into a recovery home, treatment center, or hospital unit for two weeks, thirty days, six months, or a year or more, to learn to live without drugs and alcohol, deliver healthy children, and have a safe place to recover. Homeless addicted women and pregnant moms are often given priority for a bed since a delay in treatment could mean more problems, especially for babies growing prenatally. The majority of hospital chemical dependency programs are not set up to have children along while a parent gets substance abuse treatment, but many hospitals do have special women's programs.

Treatment programs that have been designed especially for women or with women and children in mind are better equipped to meet the complex and consuming needs of women, children, and their addiction issues. People who work in women's programs usually have hopeful, positive attitudes about addicted moms and affected children, which is a strong motivator for a woman's lasting recovery. They are familiar with family-oriented community services, female abuse issues, childcare matters, parenting techniques, economic realities, and relationship problems common to women and mothers everywhere.

Just like in school, men tend to dominate the conversation when men and women are in the same treatment groups. Men frequently outnumber women in coed programs, and often women don't speak up as much when guys are around. Since addiction influences the lives of men and women differently, the methods of treating women's substance abuse should also be different.

Stereotyping, blaming, and double standards occur less frequently in a supportive female environment. When women come to terms with their drug and alcohol addictions, depression, low self-worth, and a lack of self-confidence can be overwhelming. Besides, it's easier for women to talk about their feelings and their problems with other women, to risk "not looking good." Telling the truth about what your life was like when you were actively using drugs and alcohol is crucial to recovery. Having to hold up a false front wouldn't help any woman toward seeing her addiction clearly, or claiming her successes as her own.

It's nice to feel safe and protected in a live-in treatment program while learning new ways to cope with problems that have been in your life a long time. We know that children require tons of attention from their caretakers, that substances are highly addictive, and that healing from intimacy, sexuality, and abuse issues can be fairly exhausting. Sometimes a drug- and alcohol-addicted woman needs all her available energy for recovery and for working on very personal matters. She should give herself all the time she needs for a more complete recovery, and the best chance at a wonderful, long life with her kids.

If your children are being cared for by somebody else, or your family or trusted friend can look after them for a short time, you may choose to go into a residential treatment program solo. This is a good option because live-in programs for women can usually be completed in less time than treatment programs or recovery homes that allow children into treatment with mom. You will then be able to rejoin your kids clean and sober, feeling more confident with new recovery skills, and better prepared for parenting.

Perinatal drug and alcohol treatment programs are generally recommended for pregnant women and mothers because they understand the many emotional, social, housing, educational, and medical needs of women and their children. Perinatal treatment workers support women in organizing family services for healthy babies and growing children. There are residential recovery homes and day care outpatient programs where moms and children receive treatment together. Some programs can work with pregnant women, some with moms and infants only, some accept kids under five years of age, while others allow children up to age fifteen. Let your fingers do the walking, call, and get the 4-1-1.

Treatment centers that work with mothers and children have many important features, such as a nursery, toddler area, fenced play-yard, prenatal classes, parenting education, childcare workers (babysitters), safety procedures, and maybe professionals who give babies and other children developmental checkups. Child specialists make sure that infants and kids are learning and growing normally, and give them extra help, if they need it.

Professionals who treat recovering mothers can help a woman maintain her self-esteem, self-worth, and her sobriety as she interacts with difficult state systems and trying family members. Feeling understood and supported by her treatment counselor, a parenting woman can keep her patience and her head afloat while struggling through these troubled waters. This is especially true if a substance abusing woman has been in treatment before, had prior cases with county agencies, or suffered mistreatment from authority figures in the past.

Moms spend a lot of time with their children in perinatal day care and residential programs, but are also given breaks from caretaking responsibilities. Women in treatment need to learn about addiction to mind-bending chemicals, new ways to cope with daily tasks, communication skills, and how to participate in adult recovery activities. Learning to have fun with children and adults, while newly clean and sober, is normally part of the treatment program, too.

After calling a treatment program for services, you may be told there is a waiting list. Don't freak out! Sadly, there are often more women and children in trouble than there are special programs to treat them. Just ask the program's intake people what they would like you to do in order to enroll. Go down for an interview, call them everyday, or do whatever is needed to move you along the list. Counselors will be more likely to work with a woman who follows direction, calling when asked to, than with someone who is flaking out and unable to show up or call. The crystal ball says that you will find your place in a recovery program. Just hang in there, and follow through. Good things are in store for you.

## Outpatient Programs

There are basic outpatient programs in most communities that are privately and publicly funded. Outpatient treatment programs that aren't specifically for women and children are for adults only, or for adolescents only. These programs generally treat men and women together, require less time, and have fewer services available for families at the treatment site. Most alcoholics and addicts in a formal program are enrolled in outpatient treatment. If you have children, however, it can be tough to get childcare, attend treatment groups in the evening, or obtain social services . . . and nobody gets well if they can't make it to their program.

While searching for a treatment program, look at outpatient programs very carefully, because some facilities meet with chemically dependent people for only a few hours every week. This amount of time for treating the disease of addiction is frequently not enough for women to make the kind of improvements they want to make in their lives. The winner's circle of recovering women and men who went to a treatment center:

- stayed at least three months or more

- received about nine hours or more of treatment every week (if in an outpatient program)

- found a caring treatment counselor they could relate to

You can find the people and the programs who can give you the recovery skills that will work for you. I know there is a winner inside of you. You won't have to recycle drugs and alcohol through your body, or let the disease of addiction attack your children ever again.

If people don't get the right kind of treatment, the right amount of help, and the best support to stay clean and sober, then next week, next month, or next year, they will need chemical dependency treatment again. Relapse into using and drinking can happen all too quickly for the people who haven't developed a personal recovery program inside their guts and in their hearts. They will not know how to stay clean and sober if life becomes stressful, or if booze and drugs are around, and we know there's a lot more to it than just saying "no."

## Twelve-Step Programs

Are you sick and tired of being sick and tired? Do you have a "nudge from the judge"? Have drugs and alcohol left you feeling worthless, betrayed, and demoralized? Good, there's hope. Millions of people, all over the world, have gotten clean and sober and stay that way from participating in a fellowship of recovering addicts and alcoholics.

Alcoholics Anonymous (AA), Narcotics Anonymous (NA), and other self-help twelve-step groups have meetings where people help each other stay clean and sober. There's power in numbers. Women, men, even doctors, lawyers, and Indian chiefs, come together in AA and NA for a common goal—sobriety. Hearing the trials and tribulations of others' lives when they were drinking and using, understanding the misery, and enjoying the humor of their story, goes a long way toward helping others believe that they, too, can recover. You will find the healing compassion that others can give through sharing experiences with life and addictive disease. People in these fellowships feel cared about and supported while using the AA and NA tools of recovery. They watch their lives, and the lives of others, get better.

A program for living is suggested that helps alcoholics and addicts with the emotional, mental, and spiritual aspects of their lives that have been deeply scarred from their dependency upon chemicals. Sometimes recovering women and men ask another AA or NA member to help them individually, and this special person becomes their sponsor. Sponsors don't tell you what to do with your life. They agree to help you in your journey of recovery, so that you can make your own good choices, and maintain and enjoy your sobriety.

The AA and NA fellowships are well-respected. Counselors, doctors, and civil and criminal court judges often ask the substance abusers they see to attend AA and NA meetings as part of their aftercare treatment plan, ongoing healthcare, or sentence. Everybody is welcomed at self-help groups, which can have meetings morning, noon, and night.

AA and NA meetings are free; nobody takes roll for attendance, there's no president or authority, no tests, and no demands. Everything is organized on a volunteer basis, and groups can be found in almost every community. There are special AA and NA meetings for women only, men only, young people, older people, lesbian and gay persons, artists, and some even have childcare. Meetings can be on specific recovery topics, have speakers only, group participation, or all of the above. You can take your pick, and talk only if you want to, but check it out no matter what.

The laughter, companionship, and warm support found in twelve-step meetings insure that recovering people will find an effective, fun substitute for drinking alcohol and using drugs. Clean and sober addicts and alcoholics insist on enjoying life, and can show you how to make the most of your recovery. All you need is honesty, an open mind, and a willingness to try.

Alcoholic beverages are shown in almost every magazine, as well as in many TV commercials, billboards, movies, and store shelves. Drugs can be found on most street corners, and inside many families, too. Regular meetings and contact with clean and sober friends met through AA and NA can be powerful protection against these pressures. Self-help groups and twelve-step meetings are recommended for women to continue living drug-free and alcohol-free, during and after their participation in a treatment program.

## Reach Out to Feel Good

Put together your very own team to help you, play-by-play, day-by-day, recover your life from alcohol and drugs. You are the star player, so let the people in your support system coach you around the danger zones and cheer you across the finish line.

Your team should include your children, treatment counselor, twelve-step sponsor, healthcare professionals, babysitters, and clean and sober people. If you are involved with state agencies, your children's social worker, probation officer, or other personnel would be members of your team. Perhaps you have a family member, minister, priest, rabbi, or other advisor, who can be there for you, too. The people you choose to be in your life, and even a few you didn't choose, can make all the difference between success or failure as you approach the goalposts, carrying the ball for a healthier family.

There is a huge community of recovering people offering their hands and their hearts to you. Completion of a treatment program will provide addicted women with a strong foundation for a new life, free of drugs and alcohol. Children become reunited with mothers who know how to lovingly and competently parent them. No longer will you need to feel ashamed or afraid because you are drunk or loaded.

Feeling good about who you are, being clean and sober, and making a brighter, better world for your children is a beautiful accomplishment. Having a purpose in life and being excited about living, are icing on the cake of recovery. Women who have changed, and escaped the ongoing pain of active alcoholism and drug addiction, will be having their cake and eating it too, for a long, long time. There's enough for everyone and anyone who is ready to recover.

You can follow the recipe for recovery, and be loved, admired, and respected for turning your life around to one of inner growth and outer success. You will also be introduced to a new person—YOU! Now that is someone worth meeting, knowing, and loving. You will have succeeded. And I am proud of you, wishing so much love to you and to your children.

## *Success*

To laugh often and much; to win the respect
of intelligent people and the affection of children; to
earn the appreciation of honest critics and endure
the betrayal of false friends; to appreciate beauty,
to find the best in others; to leave the world a bit
better, whether by a healthy child, a garden patch,
or a redeemed social condition; to know even one
life has breathed easier because you have lived.
This is to have succeeded.

Ralph Waldo Emerson

# CHAPTER 9

# Referrals:
# People to Call, Info to Get
# (and It's Free!)

## Drug and Alcohol Treatment and Self-Help Groups

Al Anon & Al Ateen Family Groups
1-800-356-9996
1-800-344-2666

Alcohol, Drugs, & Pregnancy Helpline
1-800-638-BABY
1-800-638-2229
1-312-541-1272

Alcohol Hotline
1-800-ALCOHOL
1-800-252-6465

Alcoholics Anonymous & Narcotics Anonymous
(call your operator for the local number in your area)

American Council for Drug Education
1-800-488-3784

American Council on Alcoholism
1-800-527-5344

Be Sober Referral Line
1-800-BE SOBER
1-800-237-6237

Betty Ford Center Referral Line
1-800-854-9211

Ceia Webb (treatment referrals for Eastern United States)
1-800-743-2342

Children of Alcoholics Foundation
1-800-359-2623

Choiceline (treatment, shelters, mental health, rape crisis, eating
disorders referrals)
1-800-824-6423

Coalition on Alcohol and Drug Dependent Women and Their
Children
1-202-737-8122

Cocaine Hotline
1-800-COCAINE
1-800-262-2463

Marijuana Anonymous World Service Office
1-800-766-6779

National Association for the Dually Diagnosed (substance abuse and mental illness)
1-800-331-5362

National Association for Native American Children of Alcoholics
1-800-322-5601

National Clearinghouse for Alcohol and Drug Information
1-800-729-6686

National Council on Alcoholism and Drug Dependence Hopeline
1-800-NCA-CALL
1-800-622-2255

National Drug and Alcohol and Treatment Information Line
1-800-662-HELP
1-800-662-4357
Spanish:  1-800-662-9832
TDD:  1-800-228-0427

National Women's Resource Center for the Prevention of Perinatal Abuse of Alcohol and Other Drugs
1-800-354-8824

PRIDE Institute Helpline (substance abuse & materials; adolescent, gay/lesbian issues)
1-800-547-7433

Primary Health (outpatient treatment and mental health)
1-800-486-9870

Recovery Options (treatment referrals for Western United States)
1-800-662-2873

United Way of America (look in your phone book's yellow pages or call the operator for local number—for substance abuse treatment and other family support services)

# Children's Safety—Save A Child and Don't Wait

Childhelp USA/ National Child Abuse Hotline
1-800-4A-CHILD
1-800-422-4453

Child Find of America, Inc.
1-800-I AM LOST
1-800-426-5678
1-800-A WAY OUT
1-800-292-9688

Children's Defense Fund
1-800-CDF-1200
1-800-233-1200

Children's Rights Foundation
1-800-329-5437

Find the Children
1-800-456-6150

Missing Children Help Center
1-800-872-5437

National Center for Missing and Exploited Children
1-800-843-5678

National Child Abuse Hotline
1-800-421-0353

National Clearinghouse on Child Abuse and Neglect Information
1-800-394-3366

National Council on Child Abuse and Family Violence Helpline
1-800-222-2000

National Kid Print Program (child safety kits)
1-800-962-9202

National Resource Center on Child Abuse and Neglect
1-800-227-5242

National Runaway Hotline
1-800-231-6946

National Runaway Switchboard
1-800-621-4000

National Youth Crisis Hotline
1-800-448-4663

We Tip National Headquarters (report crimes, caller anonymous)
1-800-472-7766

## Women's Health and Safety—Don't Wait

American Liver Foundation and Hepatitis & Liver Disease Hotline
1-800-223-0179

Battered Women's Bilingual Hotline
1-800-548-2722

Best Start (breast-feeding)
1-800-277-4975

CDC Sexually Transmitted Diseases Hotline
1-800-227-8922

CDC National AIDS Information Clearinghouse
1-800-458-5231

Depression After Delivery Information Request Line
1-800-944-4773

Drug-Free Workplace Helpline
1-800-967-5752

Endometriosis Association
1-800-992-3636

Grief Recovery Helpline
1-800-445-4808

Incest Survivors Anonymous
1-310-428-5599

International Childbirth Education Association
1-800-624-4934

La Leche League International (breast-feeding)
1-800-525-3243

National Abortion Federation (safe & legal termination)
1-800-772-9100

National AIDS Information Hotline
English: 1-800-342-AIDS
or 1-800-342-2437
Spanish: 1-800-344-SIDA
or 1-800-344-7432
Native American: 1-800-283-2437
Hearing Impaired: 1-800-553-AIDS
Multilingual/Asian Pacific: 1-800-922-2438

National Association for Sickle Cell Disease
1-800-421-8453

National Black Women's Health Project
1-202-835-0117

National Eating Disorder Hotline & Referral Service
1-800-248-3285

National Foundation for Depressive Illness (Depression) Helpline
1-800-248-4344

National Health Information Center (refers to appropriate health
organization)
1-800-336-4797

National Hospice Organization Referral Line
1-800-658-8898

National Kidney Foundation Information Center
1-800-622-9010

National Lung Line Information Service
1-800-222-LUNG
1-800-222-5864

National Mental Health Association Information
1-800-969-6642

National Mental Health Consumer Self-Help Clearinghouse
1-800-553-4539

National Organization for Breast Cancer Information Hotline
1-800-221-2141
1-312-986-8228

National Rehabilitation Information Center
1-800-346-2742

Peaceful Pregnancy (childbirth, nutrition materials)
1-800-488-7322

Planned Parenthood Federation of America
1-800-829-7732

PMS Access Info Line
1-800-222-4767

Pregnancy Counseling Services (unwed mothers to age 22)
1-800-542-4453

Prostitutes Anonymous World Service Office & Referral Center
1-402-393-0828

Rader Institute (eating disorders)
1-800-255-1818

Sexual Assault, Rape, Domestic Violence Crisis Hotline
1-800-656-4673

## Parent Support Services

Active Parenting (support groups, materials)
1-800-825-0060

Adoptive and Foster Parents of FAS and Drug-Affected Children
(support network), Bergen County Council on Alcoholism
1-201-261-1450

Allergy and Asthma Network/Mothers of Asthmatics
1-800-878-4403

American Cancer Society
1-800-227-2345

American Cleft Palate Education Foundation
1-800-242-5338

American Diabetes Association National Center
1-800-232-3472

American Foundation for the Blind Info Line
1-800-232-5463

American Heart Association
1-800-242-8721

American Red Cross (disaster relief)
1-800-540-2000

Beginnings for Parents of Hearing Impaired Children
1-800-541-HEAR
1-800-541-4327

Buckle-Up & Safety Restraint (car seat) Line
1-800-282-5587

Elder Abuse Hotline
1-800-992-1660

Epilepsy Foundation of America Patient & Family Information
Center
1-800-EFA-1000
1-800-332-1000

Family Resource Coalition (family support services in your area)
1-312-341-0900

Federal Information Center (refers to appropriate Federal Office in
your area)
1-800-688-9889

Food and Water, Inc.
1-800-EAT-SAFE
1-800-328-7233

Food Safety, USDA Meat & Poultry Hotline
1-800-535-4555

Friends of Karen (emotional, financial support for families whose
children have life-threatening illness)
1-800-637-2774

Human Growth Foundation
1-800-451-6434

Institute for Black Parenting
1-800-367-8858

Just Say No International (community prevention program)
1-800-258-2766

Juvenile Justice Clearinghouse (prostitution, delinquency, legal info)
1-800-638-8736

Make-a-Wish Foundation (terminal illness)
1-800-722-WISH
1-800-722-9474

Mothers Against Drunk Driving (substance abuse info and support for victims)
1-800-992-6233

Mothers' Centers National Association
1-800-645-3828

Mothers Without Custody
1-800-457-6962

National Association for the Dually Diagnosed (mental illness & mental retardation)
1-800-331-5362

National Association for Parents of the Visually Impaired
1-800-562-6265

Nutrition Hotline of the American Dietetic Association
1-800-366-1655

National Lead Poisoning Information Center
1-800-424-LEAD
1-800-424-5352

National Mental Health Association
1-800-433-5959

National Parent Resource Center (children with special needs)
1-800-331-0688

National Rehabilitation Information Center
1-800-346-2742

National Resource Center on Homelessness and Mental Illness
1-800-444-7415

National Safety Council Call Center (home safety)
1-800-621-7619

National SIDS (Sudden Infant Death Syndrome) Alliance Helpline
1-800-221-7437

Office of Minority Health Resource Center
1-800-444-6472

Parents Against Cancer Together Support Group
1-800-962-4748

Parents Anonymous (call operator for your local number)

Parents Without Partners (support meetings & children's activities)
1-800-637-7974

Pesticides Advice Network
1-800-858-7378

Poison Control Center Hotline (call your operator for local 24-hour number)

Resident Initiatives (HUD) Clearinghouse
1-800-955-2232

Scoliosis Association
1-800-800-0669

Single Parent Resource Center
1-212-988-0991

ToughLove International
1-800-333-1069

Welfare Mother's Voice
1-414-444-0220

## Support Services for Children

American Association on Mental Retardation
1-800-424-3688

American Society for Deaf Children
1-800-942-ASDC
1-800-942-2732

American Speech-Language-Hearing Association Information
Resource Center
1-800-638-8255

Asthma and Allergy Foundation of America Information Clearinghouse
1-800-7-ASTHMA
1-800-727-8462

Blind Children's Center
1-800-222-3567

Candlelighters Childhood Cancer Foundation
1-800-366-2223

Child Care Aware, National Association of Childcare Resources
and Referral Agencies
1-800-424-2246

Children's Craniofacial Association (facial disfigurement)
1-800-535-3643

Children's Hospice International
1-800-24-CHILD
1-800-242-4453

Clearinghouse on Disabilities and Gifted Education (for children)
1-800-328-0272

Council for Exceptional Children (disabled & gifted children)
1-800-845-6232

Federation for Children with Special Needs
1-800-331-0688

Head Start County Childcare Program (call operator for local number)

Juvenile Diabetes Foundation International
1-800-223-1138

Learning Disabilities Association of Washington (learning disabilities and attention deficit disorder)
1-206-882-0792

National Alliance for the Mentally Ill Helpline
1-800-950-6264

National Center for Stuttering
1-800-221-2483

National Down Syndrome Society
1-800-232-6372
1-800-221-4602

National Information Center for Children and Youth with Disabilities
1-800-695-0285

National Information Clearinghouse for Infants with Disabilities and Life-Threatening Conditions
1-800-922-1107, X201
1-800-922-9234, X201

National Pediatric HIV Resource Center
1-800-362-0071

National Rainbow Coalition (program for African-American youth, ages 8–18)
1-202-728-1180

National Youth Crisis Hotline (counseling and summer camps)
1-800-HIT HOME
1-800-448-4663

Orton Dyslexia Society (learning disabilities)
1-800-222-3123

Pathways Awareness Foundation (physical movement delays)
1-800-955-2445

Scott Newman Center, America Belongs to Our Children
1-800-783-6396

Spina Bifida Association of America
1-800-621-3141

Starting Point Child Care Resource & Referral Service
1-800-880-0971

United Way Childcare Program (call operator for local number)

YMCA and YWCA Childcare Programs (call operator for local numbers)

# Books and Magazines for Kids and Moms

American Library Association
1-800-545-2433

Chinaberry Book Service (children's books by mail)
1-800-776-2242

Imprints (newsletter of the Birth and Life Parenting Issues
Bookstore)
1-800-736-0631

New Harbinger Publications, Inc. (for copies of this guide)
1-800-748-6273

Single Mother (magazine of National Organization of Single
Mothers—call for free back issues)
1-704-888-KIDS
1-704-888-5437

Twins (magazine for multiple births)
1-800-821-5533

Waterfront Books for Kids and Parents
1-800-639-6063

# Appendix

## American Society of Addiction Medicine, Inc.

*Public Policy Statement on Chemically
Dependent Women and Pregnancy*

## Background

Because of the adverse effects on fetal development of alcohol and certain other drugs (including nicotine, cocaine, marijuana, and opiates) the chemically dependent woman who is pregnant or may become pregnant is an especially important candidate for intervention and treatment. Similarly, prevention programs should target all women of childbearing age.

Recently, public concern for preventing fetal harm has resulted in punitive measures against pregnant women or women in the postpartum period. These measures have included incarcerating pregnant women in jails to keep them abstinent and the criminal prosecution of mothers for taking drugs while pregnant and thereby passing these substances to the fetus or newborn through the placenta.

The American Society of Addiction Medicine is deeply committed to the prevention of alcohol and other drug-related harm to the health and well-being of children. The most humane and effective way to achieve this end is through education, intervention, and treatment. The imposition of criminal penalties solely because a person suffers from an illness is inappropriate and counterproductive. Criminal prosecution of chemically dependent women will have the overall result of deterring such women from seeking both prenatal care and chemical dependency treatment, thereby increasing, rather than preventing, harm to children and to society as a whole.

# Policy Recommendations

The American Society of Addiction Medicine supports the following policies:

1. Prevention programs to educate all members of the public about the dangers of alcohol and other drug use during pregnancy and lactation. These should include:

   • Age appropriate school-based education throughout the school curriculum.

   • Public education about alcohol and other drug use in pregnancy and lactation, including health warning labels and posters as well as radio and television messages, educational programs and written materials.

   • Prenatal education about alcohol and other drugs for all pregnant women and significant others, as part of adequate prenatal care.

   • Professional education for all healthcare professionals, including education of obstetricians and pediatricians in the care of chemically dependent women and their offspring.

2. Early intervention, consultation, and case finding programs specifically designed to reach chemically dependent women:

  - Screening for alcohol and other drug problems in all obstetric care services, as well as in all medical settings.

  - Adequate case finding, intervention, and referral services for women identified as suffering from chemical dependency.

3. Treatment services able to meet the needs of chemically dependent women:

  - Appropriate and accessible chemical dependency treatment services for pregnant women and women of childbearing age and their families, including inpatient and residential treatment. Services to care for the children and newborns of these patients should be provided. Without adequate child care arrangements, chemically dependent women are often unable to engage in the treatment they need.

  - Adequate facilities for the outpatient and aftercare phases of treatment for chemically dependent women.

  - Adequate perinatal care for chemically dependent women in treatment, sensitive to their special needs.

  - Adequate child protection services to provide alternative placement for infants or children of persons suffering from chemical dependency who are unable to function as parents, in the absence of others able to fulfill the parent role.

4. Research:

  - Basic and clinical research on the effects of alcohol and other drugs used during pregnancy.

  - Model programs, with evaluation component, for case finding, intervention and treatment of chemically dependent pregnant women, and for case finding, intervention, and treatment of infants and children affected by maternal alcohol and/or other drug use.

5. Law enforcement:

- State and local governments should avoid any measures defining alcohol or other drug use during pregnancy as "prenatal child abuse," and should avoid prosecution, jail, or other punitive measures as a substitute for providing effective health services for these women.

6. Preservation of patient confidentiality:

- No law or regulation should require physicians to violate confidentiality by reporting their pregnant patients to state or local authorities for "prenatal child abuse."

*Adopted by ASAM Board of Directors 9/25/89*

# Bibliography

## Chapter 1

American College of Obstetricians and Gynecologists. 1994. ACOG Technical Bulletins 194 and 195 Washington, DC: ACOG.

American Health Consultants. 1991. "Drug-abusing women provide family planning challenge." *Contraceptive Technology Update* 12(2): 17–32.

Information Plus. 1993. *Illegal Drugs and Alcohol: America's Anguish.* Wylie, TX: Information Plus.

Jessup, M. 1990. "The treatment of perinatal addiction: identification, intervention, and advocacy." *Western Journal of Medicine* 152 (5): 553–558.

National Institute on Drug Abuse. 1991. *1990 National Household Survey on Drug Abuse.* U.S. Department of Health and Human Services. Rockville, MD.

Neimark, J., Conway, C., Doskoch, P. 1994. "Back from the drink." *Psychology Today.* (9/10): 46–53.

Pleck, J.H., Sonenstein, F.L. 1995. "Warning: Our cultures direct and indirect messages about contraception are hazardous to teens' health!" Protecting Sexually Active Youth Network 3(1): 2–3.

Teets, J.M. 1990. "What women talk about: Sexuality issues of chemically dependent women." *Journal of Psychosocial Nursing* 28: 4–7.

Vega, W.A., Kolody, B., Hwang, J., Noble, A. 1993. "Prevalence and magnitude of perinatal substance exposures in California." *New England Journal of Medicine* 329:850–854.

Zabin, L.S., Astone, N.M., Emerson, M.R. 1993. "Do adolescents want babies: The relationship between attitudes and behavior." *Journal of Research on Adolescents* 3(1): 67–86.

## Chapter 2

Alcoholics Anonymous. "For women only." Los Angeles: Undated handout.

Black, C. 1981. *It Will Never Happen To Me*. Denver: M.A.C. Printing and Publishing Division.

Ewing, H. 1990. "A practical guide to intervention in health and social services with pregnant and postpartum addicts and alcoholics." *Tools for Effective Intervention*. California State Alcohol and Drug Programs. 42–48.

Jessup, M. 1990. "The treatment of perinatal addiction: Identification, intervention, and advocacy." *Western Journal of Medicine* May 152: 553–558.

Jones, J.W. 1982. CAST: Children of Alcoholics Screening Test. Family Recovery Press.

Morse, R., Flavin, D. 1992. "The definition of alcoholism." *Journal of the American Medical Association* 268, no. 8.

Pokorny, A.D., Miller, B.A., Kaplan, H.B. 1972. "The brief MAST: A shortened version of the Michigan Alcoholism Screening Test." *American Journal of Psychiatry* 129: 342–345.

The Women's Action Alliance. "Questions about prescription drug use." New York: Undated handout.

# Chapter 3

Alexander, S. 1994. *In Praise of Single Parents.* Boston: Houghton-Mifflin Company.

Cohen, J.B. 1991. "Why woman partners of drug users will continue to be at high risk for HIV infection." *Journal of Addictive Diseases* 10 no. 4.

Kellermann, J.L. 1977. "Grief: A basic reaction of alcoholism." Hazelden Foundation. Center City, MN.

Reed, B.G. 1987. "Developing women-sensitive drug dependence treatment services: Why so difficult?" *Journal of Psychoactive Drugs* 19(2): 151–163.

Schneider, J.W., Chasnoff, I.J. 1987. "Cocaine abuse during pregnancy." *Top Acute Trauma Care Rehabilitation, Inc.* 2(1): 59–69.

Tracy, C.E. 1990. "Social impact of drugs on women and children." Pennsylvania Perinatal Association. Bryn Mawr, PA.

# Chapter 4

Anthony, C.P., Kolthoff, N.J. 1971. *Textbook of Anatomy and Physiology.* St. Louis: C.V. Mosby Company.

Bobak, I.M., Jensen, M.D., Zalar, M.K. 1989. *Maternity and Gynecologic Care.* St. Louis: C.V. Mosby Company.

Cates, W., Alexander, E.R. 1988. *Sexually Transmitted Diseases and the Fetus: A Continuing Challenge.* New York: New York Academy of Sciences.

Chasnoff, I.J. 1988. "Drug use in pregnancy: Parameters at risk." *Children at Risk* 35, no. 6.

Hanna, L. 1994. *Mother-to-child HIV Transmission.* Emeryville, CA: Infocom Group.

Jessup, M. 1990. "The treatment of perinatal addiction: Identification, intervention, and advocacy." *The Western Journal of Medicine* 152: 553–558.

Mitchell, H.S., Rynbergen, H.J., Anderson, L., Dibble, M.V. 1968. *Cooper's Nutrition in Health and Disease.* 15th Ed. Philadelphia: J.B. Lippincott Company.

O'Connor, P.G., Selwyn, P.A., Schottenfeld, R.S. 1994. "Medical care for injection-drug users with human immunodeficiency virus infection." *The New England Journal of Medicine* August 18: 450–459.

Santrock, J.W. 1993. *Children.* 3rd Ed. Dubuque, IA: Brown & Benchmark Publishers.

Thomas, C.L., ed. 1974. *Taber's Cyclopedic Medical Dictionary.* 12th Ed. Philadelphia: F.A. Davis Co.

U.S. Department of Health and Human Services. "Tuberculosis facts—exposure to TB." Center for Disease Control. Atlanta, GA: No. 00–5983.

# Chapter 5

Ajuluchukwu, D.C., Brown, L.S., Crummey, F.C., Foster, K.F., Ismail, Y.I., Siddiqui, N. 1993. "Demographic, medical history and sexual correlates of HIV seropositive methadone maintained women." *Journal of Addictive Diseases* 12(4).

American Association for World Health. "Environmental tobacco smoke fact sheet for World No-Tobacco Day." Washington, DC.

American Association for World Health. "Women and tobacco fact sheet for World No-Tobacco Day." Washington, D.C.

American College of Obstetricians and Gynecologists. 1994. "Substance abuse in pregnancy." ACOG Technical Bulletin no. 195: 1–6. Washington, D.C.: ACOG

The American Council for Drug Education. 1986. "Drugs and pregnancy; it's not worth the risk."

Anthony, C.P., Kolthoff, N.J. 1971. *Textbook of Anatomy and Physiology.* St. Louis: C.V. Mosby Company.

Chasnoff, I.J. 1988. "Newborn infants with drug withdrawal symptoms." *Pediatrics in Review* 9(9): 273–278.

Chasnoff, I.J. 1991. "Cocaine and pregnancy: Clinical and methodologic issues." *Clinics in Perinatology* 18(1): 113–123.

Chasnoff, I.J, Burns, K.A., Burns, W.J., Schnoff, S.H. 1986. "Prenatal drug exposure: Effects on neonatal and infant growth and development." *Neurobehavioral Toxicology and Teratology* 8: 357–362.

Chavez, C.J., Ostrea, E.M., Stryker, J.C., Smialek, Z. 1979. "Sudden infants death syndrome among infants of drug-dependent mothers." *Journal of Pediatrics* (95): 407–409.

Chisum, G.M. 1990. "Nursing interventions with the antepartum substance abuser." *Journal of Perinatal Neonatal Nursing.* Aspen Publishers, Inc. 3(4): 26–33.

Committee on Substance Abuse and Committee on Children with Disabilities. 1993. "Fetal alcohol syndrome and fetal alcohol effects." *Pediatrics* 91(5): 1004–1005.

Inaba, D.S., Cohen, W.E. 1990. *Uppers, Downers, All Arounders: Physical and Mental Effects of Drugs of Abuse.* 3rd Ed. Ashland, OR: Cinemed Inc.

Kaltenbach, K., Silverman, N., Wapner, R. 1992. "Methadone maintenance during pregnancy." *The State Methadone Treatment Guidelines.* U.S. Department of Health and Human Services. Center for Substance Abuse Treatment. Rockville, MD: no. 91–MF358084.

National Association of Perinatal Addiction and Education. 1989. "Substances most commonly abused during pregnancy and their risk to mother and baby." Handout.

National Institute on Alcohol Abuse and Alcoholism. 1990. "Alcohol and health: Fetal alcohol syndrome and other effects of alcohol on pregnancy outcome." U.S. Department of Health and Human Services. Rockville, MD.

Zweben, J.E., Payte, J.T. 1990. "Methadone maintenance in the treatment of opioid dependence—a current perspective." *Western Journal of Medicine* 152 (May): 588–599.

## Chapter 6

Alcoholics Anonymous World Services, Inc. 1976. *"Alcoholics Anonymous: The story of how many thousands of men and women have recovered from alcoholism."* New York: Alcoholics Anonymous.

American Civil Liberties Union. "Infant victims of drug abuse." U.S. Senate Hearing, Committee on Finance. Washington, D.C. June 28, 1990.

Bolane, J.E. 1991. *Birth Companion: A Guide for Support During Labor and Birth.* Rochester, NY: Childbirth Graphics Ltd.

The Boston Women's Health Book Collective. 1984. *The New Our Bodies, Ourselves.* New York: Simon and Schuster and Touchstone.

Committee on Substance Abuse. 1990. "Drug exposed infants." *Pediatrics* 86(4): 639–642.

Durfee, M., Tilton-Durfee, D. 1990. "Interagency intervention with perinatal substance abuse." *Children Today.* (7–8): 30–32.

English, A. 1990. "Prenatal drug exposure: Grounds for mandatory child abuse reports?" *Youth Law News* 11(1): 3–8.

Griffith, D.R. 1989. "Neurobehavioral effects of intrauterine cocaine exposure." *Ab Initio: An International Newsletter for Professionals Working with Infants and Their Families* 1(1).

Information Plus. 1993. *Illegal Drugs and Alcohol: America's Anguish.* Wylie, TX: Information Plus.

Institute of Medicine. 1985. "Preventing low birthweight summary." Washington, DC: National Academy Press.

Kaufman, G. 1992. *Shame: The Power of Caring.* 3rd Ed. Rochester, VT: Schenkman Books, Inc.

Kelly, M., Parsons, E. 1992. *The Mother's Almanac.* New York: Doubleday.

Logli, P.A. 1992. "The prosecutor's role in solving the problems of prenatal drug use and substance exposed children." *Hastings Law Journal* San Francisco: 43, no. 3.

Lorde, A. 1984. *Sister Outsider.* Trumansburg, NY: The Crossing Press Feminist Series.

Los Angeles County Department of Children's Services. 1986. "What's happening to me? A guide to dependency court proceedings." Department of Children's Services, Juvenile Court Services. Los Angeles, CA (January).

Marshall, A.B. 1995. "Families, addiction research and education update." *The National Association For Families and Addiction Research and Education. 1994 Legislative Update.* Chicago.

National Council of Juvenile and Family Court Judges: Permanency Planning for Children Project. 1992. "Protocol for making reasonable efforts to preserve families in drug-related dependency cases." Reno, NV.

Office of National Drug Control Policy. 1993. "Breaking the cycle of drug abuse: 1993 Interim National Drug Control Strategy."

Sturner, W.Q., et al. 1991. "Cocaine babies: The scourge of the 90s." *Journal of Forensic Science* 36: 34–37.

Tucker, M.O. 1994. "Memorandum to all hospital administrators and staff." Juvenile Division, The Superior Court of California. Re: Minimum protocols for response to births involving indications of prenatal substance abuse.

# Chapter 7

Battle, J., Payne, K., Wilson, M.S. 1994. *The Open Arms Baby Book: Special Care Techniques for Infants Prenatally Exposed to Drugs or Alcohol.* Pasadena, CA: Open Arms Family Support Network.

Best, L.C. 1993. *Guiding Our Children Beyond Risk: A Handbook for Prenatally Drug-Exposed Children.* 2nd Ed. San Francisco: The Clearinghouse for Drug Exposed Children.

Childhood Injury Prevention Project. 1993. *Safety . . . For Your Child's Sake: Birth to Six Months.* San Marcos, CA: North County Health Services.

Drehobl, K.F., Fuhr, M.G. 1991. *Pediatric Massage for the Child with Special Needs.* Tucson, AZ: Therapy Skill Builders.

Educational Programs, Inc. 1994. *Guide for Expectant Parents.* 2nd Issue. Elkins Park, PA: Educational Programs, Inc.

Fine, L. 1990. *Normal Sleep Patterns: Healthy Kids Birth–3.* New York: Cahners Publishing Co.

Honig, A.S. 1989. *Love & Learn: Discipline for Young Children.* Washington, D.C.: National Association for the Education of Young Children.

Kaiser Permanente Medical Care Program. 1990. "About speech and language disorders." South Deerfield, MA: Channing L. Bete Co., Inc.

Kelly, M., Parsons, E. 1992. *The Mother's Almanac, Revised.* New York: Doubleday.

Kimmel, M.M., Segel, E. 1988. *For Reading Out Loud! A Guide to Sharing Books With Children.* New York: Delacorte Press.

Poulsen, M.K. 1992. "Perinatal substance abuse: What's best for the children?" Executive Summary Report. State of California Child Development Programs Advisory Committee. Sacramento, CA.

Ross Laboratories. 1987. *You and Your Baby: The Phenomena of Early Development.* Columbus, Ohio: Ross Laboratories.

Santrock, J.W. 1993. *Children.* 3rd Edition. Brown & Benchmark. Dubuque, IA.

Schneider, J.W., Griffith, D.R., Chasnoff, I.J. 1989. "Infants exposed to cocaine in utero: Implications for developmental assessment and intervention." *Infants and Young Children*. 2(1): 25–36.

UCLA Infant and Family Services Program. "Special care for special babies." UCLA Intervention Program. Grant No. 024AH50027.

White, E. 1992. "Foster parenting the drug-affected baby." *Zero to Three* 13(1): 13–17.

Zuckerman, B. 1991. "Drug-exposed infants: understanding the medical risk." *The Future of Children*. Spring: 26–35.

# Chapter 8

Alcoholics Anonymous World Services, Inc. 1976. *"Alcoholics Anonymous: The story of how many thousands of men and women have recovered from alcoholism."* New York: Alcoholics Anonymous.

Chasnoff, I.J. 1986. *Drug Use in Pregnancy: Mother and Child.* Norwell, MA: MTP Press of Kluwer Academic Publishers.

Chasnoff, I.J. 1989. *Drugs, Alcohol, Pregnancy and Parenting.* Lancaster, UK: Kluwer Academic Publishers.

Department of Health and Social Services. 1994. "State resources and services related to alcohol and other drug problems." National Institute of Drug Abuse. Rockville, MD.

Institute for Health Policy, Brandeis University. 1993. "Substance abuse: The nation's number one health problem; key indicators for policy." The Robert Wood Johnson Foundation. Princeton, NJ.

Kandall, S.R., Chavkin, W. 1992. "Illicit drugs in America: History, impact, on women and infants, and treatment strategies for women." *Hastings Law Journal*. 43.

Nunes-Dinis, M., Barth, R.P. 1993. "Cocaine treatment and outcome." *Social Work*. 38, no. 5.

Rawson, R., Ling, W. 1991. "Opioid addiction treatment modalities and some guidelines for their optimal use." *Journal of Psychoactive Drugs.* 23(2).

Reed, B.G. 1987. "Developing women-sensitive drug dependence treatment services: Why so difficult?" *Journal of Psychoactive Drugs* 19(2): 151–164.

R.O.W. Sciences, Inc. 1992. "Helping homeless people with alcohol and other drug problems: A guide for service providers." National Institute of Alcohol Abuse and Alcoholism. U.S. Department of Health and Human Services. Rockville, MD.

Tittle, B., St. Claire, N. 1989. "Promoting the health and development of drug-exposed infants through a comprehensive clinic model." *Zero to Three.* 18–20.

Weiner, L., Morse, B.A. 1988. *"FAS: Clinical perspectives and prevention. Drugs, Alcohol, Pregnancy, and Parenting."* Lancaster, UK: Kluwer Academic Publishers.

# Chapter 9

Pickett, O.K., Clark, E.M., Kavanagh, L.D., Eds. 1994. *Reaching Out: A Directory of National Organizations Related to Maternal and Child Health.* Arlington, VA: National Center for Education in Maternal and Child Health.

National Healthlines Directory. 1992. Arlington, VA: Information Resources Press, a division of Herner and Company.

Riddick-Norton, G. 1990. *Social Service Resource Directory for Los Angeles County 1991-1992.* Newport Beach, CA: Graphic Publishers.

# Other New Harbinger Self-Help Titles

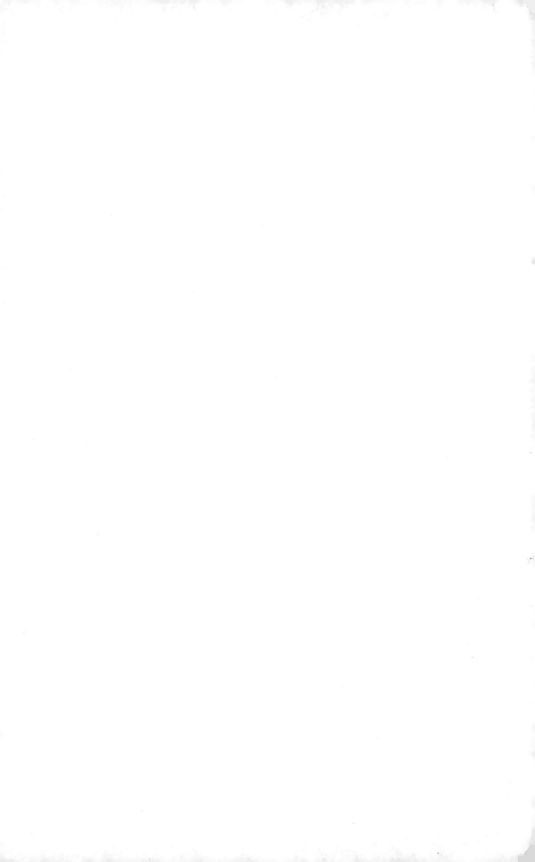

1-64794
may